THE Traveler's MEDICAL MANUAL

Geraldine Marie -

For once I thought I'd write a poem,
That other folks can read.
When the words will not reveal,
Some personal fact or deed.
This work may not be great,
Nor will it bring me fame.
But for all the parts you played,
I thank you just the same.
First was my trip to amazon,
When I began to read,
Of all the ills and dangers,
Of which I should take heed.
Then came the LDB book,
Which you told me to write.
And then a course on publishing,
Where you sent me at night.
Not to mention typing and reading every word,
And spelling diarrhea to some ~~would~~ seem absurd.
Now for trips to bookstores,
To help arrange display.
I thank you for this manual
That's on the shelves today.

Your loving husband
Me

THE Traveler's MEDICAL MANUAL

By Angelo T. Scotti, M.D.
with Thomas A. Moore

BERKLEY BOOKS, NEW YORK

This book is intended to be your guide to healthy travelling. Your physician can best decide which prescription drugs are right for you. Be sure to consult your doctor before planning a trip abroad, and read the labels on over-the-counter products carefully. Remember, nothing replaces good common sense.

To my wife, Geraldine, the best traveler in our family. Her quiet strength and inspiration encourage me to accomplish many things.

Grateful acknowledgment is made to
The International Association for Medical Assistance to Travellers (IAMAT)
for permission to reprint the IAMAT Directory of Physicians and the maps found on pages 79 and 104.

THE TRAVELER'S MEDICAL MANUAL

A Berkley Book/published by arrangement with the author

PRINTING HISTORY
Berkley trade paperback edition/June 1985

For information address: The Berkley Publishing Group, 200 Madison Avenue, New York, New York 10016.

ISBN: 0-425-07758-6

A BERKLEY BOOK ® TM 757,375

PRINTED IN THE UNITED STATES OF AMERICA

ACKNOWLEDGMENTS

I wish to thank Dr. Vincenzo Marcolongo for allowing us to use material prepared by the excellent organization which he created, the International Association for Medical Assistance to Travellers (IAMAT).

Additional thanks go to Mary Moore, Geraldine Scotti, Ellie Shepard and Joan Vossen for their assistance in preparing this manuscript.

Broad, wholesome, charitable views of men and things cannot be acquired by vegetating on one little corner of the earth all one's lifetime.

Mark Twain,
Innocents Abroad, Vol. II

CONTENTS

INTRODUCTION

Each year millions of Americans enjoy the pleasures of travel. Vacation and business trips take these travelers throughout the United States and to many foreign countries. Traveling can be great fun and provide an educational experience, but it is also very demanding. It will tax your physical and emotional reserves, and if you expect to enjoy your trip, you must anticipate and be able to handle the extra stresses and demands. For those who are not prepared, the enjoyment of a vacation or the accomplishments of a business trip may be overshadowed by a medical emergency.

Anticipation of and consideration of ways to avoid possible illnesses or injuries are the most effective means of preventing them. Travelers who are aware that they risk contracting specific illnesses in a country on their itinerary can protect themselves by obtaining the proper immunizations before embarking on their journey. If travelers are aware of the possible dangers of eating raw shellfish while away from home, they can prevent a bout of typhoid, cholera, or hepatitis. And smart travelers have discovered that carrying a first-aid kit equipped with certain prophylactic medications can save a trip that might have been ruined by such problems as seasickness or traveler's diarrhea. Unfortunately, not all health problems that occur while traveling can be prevented. For those, the abilities to recognize the early signs of illnesses and to deal with certain health emergencies until medical attention can be sought are extremely important.

This manual contains specific information for use before, during, and after your trip. The best way to use this book is to read the table of contents and familiarize yourself with the topics. When planning a trip, refer to the appropriate topics and check the worldwide directory in this book for the locations you will visit. This approach will help you make any special preparations recommended for visitors to your destination. At the very least, take this manual with you and simply refer to the table of contents if medical problems arise.

A discussion with your physician before you depart will

help you maintain good health during your trip. Remember that some illnesses contracted while traveling may not become clinically apparent for a considerable length of time. Therefore, if a new problem should arise after you return home, be sure to inform your physician of your recent travels.

A little extra effort can make your trip as safe and comfortable as your day-to-day life at home. After all, almost every place you visit is home for people who live an enjoyable life there. If you are prepared, you will have the advantage of the fresh enjoyment which comes from the unfamiliar. One person's routine environment is another's new adventure.

Bon voyage!

Prevention and Preparation

Typhoid fever, viral hepatitis, polio and malaria are among the many communicable diseases and infections which occur worldwide. The risks of contracting any of these illnesses varies with the area you visit and your immune status. Although certain diseases are consistently endemic to specific areas, the situation can change suddenly and unpredictably. Therefore, travelers should adopt as many protective measures as possible.

Travelers in the United States and in Canada, Australia, Europe, and New Zealand run a lower risk of illness than travelers in certain areas of Asia, Africa, South America, Central America, Mexico, the Middle East, and the Far East. Generally, cities, and the usual tourist areas, are not as dangerous as rural and infrequently visited locations. However, if you let your guard down, you may by exposed to disease and subsequently become ill in any country in the world.

Before you depart, check your health record and bring your immunization status up-to-date. The usual vaccinations should include those for polio, rubella, mumps, measles, tetanus, and diphtheria. After you've done this, check the requirements for the countries you intend to visit to determine if additional measures, such as immunoglobulin shots or vaccines against cholera, plague, rabies, typhoid, typhus, and yellow fever are in order.

Make an appointment with your physician to discuss your trip and to get additional vaccines if needed. Try to visit your doctor approximately one month before your trip so that sufficient time is available to receive all necessary vaccines. Ask your doctor for any prescriptions you may need while traveling. Obtain at least twice the amount of medication that you are likely to need. Carry half of it with you and pack the other half separately. Also obtain any necessary prescriptions and medication you'll want to take along in the medical kit recommended on page 5. Also obtain any necessary prescriptions and medications you'll want to take along in a medical kit (see *A Traveler's Medical Kit*).

Most of the serious illnesses that could affect you while traveling are transmitted by insects or by contaminated food or drink. Use insect repellent where malaria, yellow fever, or dengue fever are present. Limit your exposure in these areas. Wear long-sleeved shirts and long pants, use mosquito netting and stay indoors during the insect-feeding periods to add to your comfort and safety. The natives of tropical areas can usually tell you what time of day or night the insects are most aggressive.

If you are traveling in Asia, Africa, South America, Central America, Mexico, the Middle East or the Far East, assume that the water and all it touches is contaminated. Even in relatively well-developed countries the drinking water may be contaminated, especially during natural and manmade disasters.

Safety rules concerning food and drink are simple to remember and very effective. Drink only boiled water, hot liquids or commercially bottled beverages, especially those containing alcohol, for they are usually safe. Contaminated water and foods washed with it constitute the greatest danger. Salads, raw vegetables and fruit, ice, drinking water, and foods eaten with the hands, such as nuts, are frequent sources of diarrhea. Eat only hot, recently cooked food. Brushing your teeth with contaminated water or putting your fingers in your mouth are subtle sources of infection commonly overlooked.

In areas such as Australia, New Zealand, and Bermuda, the risk of acquiring an infection from contaminated food, water or drug products is generally much lower than in these locales mentioned above and is probably no greater than the risk associated with travel in the United States.

Think about the physical aspects of your trip and ask yourself whether or not you are up to it. Don't assume that you can be safely and comfortably much more active than you normally are. If you plan to carry bags, walk long distances, hike, or participate in sports or other physical activities, prepare yourself. Test yourself before you embark and gradually increase the appropriate activities until you can perform comfortably at the level necessary for travel. Better yet, begin a regular exercise program to condition yourself and continue the program during the trip and thereafter.

If for some reason you find that you cannot physically tolerate the necessary level of function, review your travel plans and revise them appropriately. It is better to know your level of ability and postpone, cancel or revise travel plans rather than ruin an expensive and time-consuming trip.

Your mental state and attitude are also quite important. Approach each trip with a positive attitude and accept the challenge of travel. As with most tasks, the benefit you receive will depend on the effort you expend. Use this manual. It will help you enjoy many miles of safe and exciting travel.

CHECKLIST

1. List of countries with required and recommended vaccines and/or precautions (see pp 105–183).
2. Medic Alert bracelet or necklace (see Medic Alert Foundation International).
3. Medical Data Card for wallet
4. Doctor's visit for discussion, prescriptions, advice, referrals, vaccines, gamma-globulin shots
5. IAMAT membership card and materials
6. Insurance cards and numbers
7. Test of physical ability to travel
8. First-aid book
9. Traveler's medical kit

MEDICAL KIT

A compact medical kit should be part of every traveler's baggage. First and foremost, your medical kit should contain any medications you need to take on a regular basis. Ask your doctor for extra prescriptions and take his or her advice concerning dosages of medications and any other items you need to include.

The medical-kit items below will help you treat most minor health problems. Check and update the contents of your kit before each trip.

PRESCRIPTION MEDICATIONS
(Consult your doctor about each.)

Codeine with acetaminophen—pain killer, cough suppressant; Standard dosage: one every 4 to 6 hours as needed

Keflex—antibiotic, for infection of skin, respiratory tract, urine; 500 mg, 4 times each day

Vistaril—antihistamine, for motion sickness, tension, nausea, insomnia; 25 mg, 4 times each day as needed

Bactrim or Septra (trimethoprim-sulfamethoxazole)—antimicrobial, for treating diarrhea or urinary infections; one twice each day.

Vibramycin (doxycycline)—antibiotic to prevent diarrhea; Standard dosage: 100 mg, each day

Silvadeen cream—for treating burns

Amoxicillin—antibiotic for sore throat, ear infection, sinus infection. Standard dosage: 500 mg, 3 times each day

Erythromycin—antibiotic for sore throat (if allergic to penicillin), lung infections. Standard dosage: 250 mg, 4 times each day

Aralen or *Fansidar (Antimalaria pills)*—if traveling to malaria-risk areas

Personal prescription medication—spare prescriptions (keep crucial ones with you)

OVER-THE-COUNTER (NONPRESCRIPTION) MEDICATIONS

Pepto-Bismol—Antacid for stomach upset; for diarrhea prevention or treatment; 1 oz. liquid or 2 chewable tablets as needed (after each loose stool)

Dramamine—antihistasmine, for motion sickness; use as directed on package

Neosporin ointment—antibiotic cream, for cuts, bruises and skin infections; apply as needed

Hydrocortisone cream—anti-inflammatory, for allergic rashes or hives

Aspirin—anti-inflammatory and pain killer

Acetaminophen (Tylenol)—pain killer

Calamine lotion—soothing lotion, for treating rashes that itch

Hydrogen peroxide—for cleaning wounds

Betadine Sticks—antiseptic, for cleansing skin

Antifungal cream or foot powder—for rashes in groin or between toes

Decongestants—Drixoral recommended, or pediatric over-the-counter medication, even for adults

SUPPLIES

Thermometer

Gauze pads (sterile)

Adhesive tape

Sling

Safety pins

Scissors

Tweezers

Soap

Insect repellent

Spare eyeglasses or contact lenses

Refraction prescription

Sunscreen

Sunglasses

Water purification tablets

Telephone numbers (your doctor's, your own)

Band-aids

Butterfly suture

Ace bandage

The Traveler's Medical Encyclopedia

AIR TRAVEL

Although air travel is one of the safest forms of transportation, flying, like any method of travel, is accompanied by the possibilities of situations not encountered at home, including fear of flying, stress, jet lag, and potential air disasters.

Most individuals can travel safely and comfortably by air, but there are others who should avoid flying or take some special precautions before boarding a plane. Those in the following categories are usually advised against traveling by air:

- Anyone who has had a *heart attack* within the last month
- Anyone with a *stroke* within the past two weeks
- Those with poorly controlled *high blood pressure*
- *Epileptics* with recent, uncontrolled seizures
- Anyone with a *wired jaw*
- Those with *severe anemia* or severe blood disorders (sickle-cell anemia, hemolytic anemia)
- *Pregnant* women *at risk* of abortion
- Women beyond their eighth month of pregnancy

Anyone with a significant medical condition that might be adversely affected by flying should discuss the traveling by air with his or her private physician. Individuals who have upper respiratory infections or allergies are more prone to the ear pain caused by pressure changes. Decongestants or cold medications taken one hour before descent may help alleviate or prevent earache. Swallowing, drinking liquids, or lightly pinching your nose shut and slowly trying to force a mouthful of air through your closed nostrils may also prevent or eliminate the pain. Babies should be given a bottle to drink during descent.

Because the air pressure in an airplane cabin is usually equivalent to that at 6500 to 8000 feet, certain lung problems may arise. Patients with severe bullous emphysema, a breathing capacity of less than 50% of normal, low blood oxygen or a high carbon-dioxide level should consult their physician before considering a trip by air. Special provisions, such as supplemental oxygen, can be provided by many airlines if they are given two day's notice. Flights at levels below 22,500 feet present fewer problems than flights at higher altitudes.

Abdominal surgery within two weeks prior to flying can cause pain and swelling of the abdomen as a result of the expansion of gas trapped therein. Patients who have recently undergone an examination of the brain called pneumoencephalography may have air trapped in the nervous system, which can likewise expand during ascent. If a traveler has gone scuba diving within twenty-four hours of a flight the ascent can cause gas bubbles in various tissues. In each of these situations, pain comes from the expansion of trapped gas. This pain is sometimes quite severe and can be relieved only by rapid descent. Therefore, individuals with any of these conditions ought to avoid flying, if possible.

Some people who are nervous about flying think that drinking an alcoholic beverage may relax them, but alcohol can cause problems for air passengers. When combined with the high altitude and dry cabin, alcohol may have a greater effect on a passenger's functional ability than it would have on the ground. Dehydration is exaggerated, and alcohol may have up to twice its usual effect.

Heart patients are not usually adversly affected by flying, but anyone with severe angina or congestive heart failure may experience chest pain and difficulty breathing. Leg swelling associated with phlebitis or varicose veins may be exacerbated by long periods of sitting. Elastic stockings and leg exercises are suggested for patients with such conditions. Periodic walks up and down the aisle are also helpful.

Disabled passengers who require wheelchairs or other assistance should notify the airlines of their special needs when making reservations so that they can be sure of accommodation. Another call to the airlines at least forty-eight hours before departure is suggested, and these passengers need to arrive at the airport at least one hour early.

Other conditions said to be aggravated by flying include asthma, cerebral vascular insufficiency, glaucoma, nasal polyps, dental cavities, abscessed teeth, colitis, peptic ulcer, and diverticulitis. However, most people with these problems can fly without difficulty. If you have any of these conditions, be sure to discuss air travel with your physician.

FEAR OF FLYING

Some people have a very real fear of flying. There are programs available which help deal with this phobia and some claim to be 90% effective. These programs are for career individuals whose jobs involve travel by air, and also for those who deprive themselves of travel because of their fear. Here is a list of some of these programs:

- Fear of Flying Clinic, 3802 Kenwood Avenue, San Mateo, CA 94403; 415-341-7595
- Flight Without Fear, P.O. Box 461, Broomfield, CO 80020; 303-398-7591 or 303-398-5829
- Fly Without Fear, 4832 Falcon Crest, Mesa, AZ 85205; 602-247-0185
- Freedom From The Fear of Flying, 2021 Country Club Prado, Coral Gables, FL 33134; 305-261-7042
- The Institute for Psychology of Air Travel, Suite 300, 25 Huntington Ave., Boston, MA 02116; 617-437-1811
- The Phobia Center of the Southwest, 12860 Hillcrest Road, Suite 119, Dallas, TX 75230; 214-386-6327
- Sprouted Wings, c/o Kathy Musman, 19026 E. Bethany Place, Aurora, CO 80013
- Tenap Program, P.O. Box 242, Northfield, NJ 08225; 609-645-7791
- Thairapy, 4500 Campus Drive, Suite 628B, Newport Beach, CA 92660; 714-641-5846

The rarest emergency is a crash landing. Use of seat belts and prompt deplaning through available exits maximizes the chances of survival in the event of a crash landing. As in all emergencies, you must remain calm, quickly evaluate your situation, and act promptly. The crew is trained to handle emergencies so listen to them and follow their instructions in such an event. If fire is present while you are in the plane, stay as close to the floor as possible, and hold your breath to avoid inhaling toxic fumes. Once out of the plane, run into the wind to avoid any flames should the airplane burn or explode. After leaving the airplane, meet in the areas designated by the crew or seek crew members for further instructions and assistance.

For additional information, see entries on *Barotrauma* and *Motion Sickness*.

EMERGENCIES IN THE AIR

Anxiety-related medical problems are among the most frequent emergencies occurring to air passengers. Hyperventilation, which is manifested by numbness in the extremities and around the lips and may be accompanied by feelings of lightheadedness or panic, can be treated by simply holding your breath as long as possible between inhalations. Other remedies include breathing into a paper bag held over your mouth and nose or counting your breaths and allowing only six to eight per minute.

Some people have found that an alcoholic drink or two before departure helps relieve their anxiety. Caffeine and other stimulants should be avoided while flying. If necessary, an antihistamine such as Vistaril may help calm passengers and will also help in preventing or treating motion sickness, another frequent malady of airline passengers.

The most common of the more serious emergencies among air travelers are seizures, heart attacks, and choking on food (aspiration). Choking most frequently occurs in people who have consumed an excessive amount of alcohol and is best treated with the Heimlich maneuver or other procedures proven to be effective for dislodging food trapped in the airway. All flight crews know the Heimlich maneuver and other life-saving techniques, but your own ability to perform them could save someone's life, even your own, in an emergency.

Individuals with seizure disorders should carry identification and medication with them and wear Medic Alert (see p. 80) emblems or some other indicator of their condition. Diabetics who are prone to hypoglycemic reactions with seizures need to carry glucagon.

Persons with heart disease should carry medication with them and report any chest pain immediately to a flight attendant. Fortunately, physicians, who may help the crew deal with significant medical emergencies, such as heart attack, are often aboard.

In spite of the availability of crew and physicians, few if any medications or instruments are available on airplanes. Therefore, anyone with unique medical problems should carry on board whatever they might need in an emergency, and they should inform a flight attendant of their potential problems.

HANDICAPPED AIRLINE PASSENGERS

The major airlines are sensitive to the unique problems of

handicapped travelers, but you must make them aware of your needs and allow them sufficient time to accommodate you. Make your reservations well in advance and state that you are handicapped and describe exactly what assistance and/or special arrangements you will need. If you intend to transport your own wheelchair, inform the representative whether or not your chair is battery-powered. If you will be accompanied by a guide dog, inform the airlines. Special equipment provided by some airlines includes wheelchairs and portable oxygen, but you must make your specific needs known in advance.

Check in earlier than normal and make your special problems and needs known to the airport and airline personnel. They will be happy to make every attempt to assist you and, if necessary, provide preboarding for you and your party.

The Airport Operators Council provides a free publication, *A Guide to Accessibility of Terminals. Access to Travel; Airports*. You may obtain this booklet by writing to Access America, Washington, D.C. 20202 or Consumer Information Center, Pueblo, Colorado 81009. It contains information on everything from parking and building facilities to restrooms and special services for the handicapped.

SPECIAL MEALS AVAILABLE ON AIRLINES

	AIRLINE						
TYPE OF MEAL	American	Braniff	Eastern	Pan Am	TWA	United	USAir
Low calorie	x	x	x	x	x	x	x
Low sodium	x	x	x	x	x	x	x
Low fat	x	x	x	x	x	x	x
Low cholesterol	x	x	x	x	x	x	x
Vegetarian	x*	x	x	x	x	x	x
Diabetic	x	x	x	x	x	x	x
Hypoglycemic			x			x	
High protein				x			
Low carbohydrate	x		x		x	x	
Gluten-free			x	x			
Bland/soft	x		x	x		x	
Kosher	x	x	x	x	x	x	x
Hindu	x**		x	x	x		
Moslem	x**		x	x	x		

* can specify if strict or lacto-ovo
**available only for certain meal flights

ALTITUDE-RELATED ILLNESSES

A number of illnesses may affect the traveler who is exposed to altitudes greater than those to which he or she is accustomed. These illnesses are related to difficulty in obtaining adequate oxygen and are caused by the lower atmospheric oxygen pressure at high altitudes. Normal healthy persons are commonly the victims of altitude sickness. Of course, individuals with heart or lung disease can expect to experience somewhat greater difficulty at higher altitudes, and they should check with their physicians before traveling to such areas.

A location of greater than 7200 feet (2000 meters) above sea level constitutes a high altitude. In order to compensate for the low oxygen levels at higher altitudes, the heart rate and the rate of respiration are increased. These changes may become apparent to the traveler within the first few days at the higher altitude.

Exertion will magnify the awareness of an increased rate of breathing and an increased heart rate. Other body systems also compensate for the low oxygen levels, resulting in changes in blood cells, kidneys and circulation. Symptoms of dysfunction may range from mild discomfort that lasts for about an hour to severe life-threatening disease that necessitates emergency therapy.

Symptoms of altitude-related illnesses may include emotional changes, lethargy, insomnia, headache, nausea, and vomiting. Breathlessness may not necessarily occur, and the absence of respiratory symptoms may mask the real nature of the problem, namely, too little oxygen.

ACUTE MOUNTAIN SICKNESS

Acute mountain sickness is characterized by nausea, headache, lethargy and difficulty sleeping during the first 48 hours after the rapid ascent to an altitude much higher than the traveler's accustomed one. The symptoms usually subside gradually during the next two days. Occasionally, more serious disease characterized by brain swelling and coma may develop.

Acute mountain sickness may be prevented by a gradual ascent to the higher altitude. If such gradual ascent is impractical for you, the administration of acetazolamide (Diamox) (Standard dosage of 125 mg to 250 mg) prior to travel and every eight hours after the commencement of travel may also help to prevent altitude sickness. Another method of preventing this problem is to take 4 mg of dexamethasone every six hours for forty-eight hours before ascent. Sedatives or sleeping medication may depress breathing, resulting in severe oxygen deprivation, and such medications should be avoided when traveling to high-altitude areas.

Rest or the administration of oxygen, or both, for a day or so may be effective in reversing acute mountain sickness. If symptoms are severe or persistent, prompt descent to a lower altitude is advisable.

HIGH-ALTITUDE PULMONARY EDEMA

High-altitude pulmonary edema may occur in anyone, but this condition is especially prevalent in young travelers who return to their high-altitude residences after a visit to a lower-altitude area. This illness usually occurs within the first forty-eight hours after arrival at altitudes above 28,000 feet (8000 meters), such as found in the Alaskan, Andes, or Himalayan mountain ranges. Lethargy, nausea, vomiting, breathlessness and coughing are the most frequent symptoms of high-altitude pulmonary edema. The skin appears blue (cyanosis), a low-grade fever may be present, and respiration may be noisy and rapid. A chest X ray will show abnormalities.

High-altitude pulmonary edema may be prevented by a slow ascent to the high-altitude area. Acetazolamide (Standard dose of 125 mg) taken prior to the ascent may also be effective. High-altitude pulmonary edema constitutes a medical emergency and medical attention must be obtained. Treatment is crucial and consists of bed rest, oxygen, and a rapid descent to a lower altitude.

HEART AND LUNG DISEASE

Pulmonary disease, such as emphysema or asthma, and heart disease may be worsened by travel to a high-altitude area or by exertion at a high altitude. Travelers with these conditions should check with their physicians before undertaking such trips and should be prepared to deal with the possible worsening of their medical problems.

To prevent the exacerbation of heart or lung disease, a gradual ascent to the higher altitude, minimal physical exertion, especially during the first few days at the higher altitude, and the prophylactic use of physician-prescribed medications are recommended.

CHRONIC MOUNTAIN SICKNESS

Chronic mountain sickness usually occurs in men and is characterized by chronic lethargy, headaches, depression or anxiety, and insomnia. This illness tends to appear in individuals who reside at high altitudes for long periods of time and is associated with polycythemia (an elevated red blood cell count). Periodic phlebotomies (bleeding) and medications such as medroxyprogesterone are two approaches to the treatment of this illness.

SUMMARY OF TREATMENT FOR ALTITUDE-RELATED ILLNESSES

1. Bedrest for the first day or two at a high altitude.
2. Gradual ascent and one or two days of rest at the new altitude to help minimize problems.
3. Prophylactic Diamox the day before travel and daily thereafter.
4. Oxygen when symptoms occur (some hotels at higher altitudes have oxygen available upon request).
5. Rapid descent to a lower altitude if other measures fail.
6. Medical care if symptoms are severe or unrelenting in spite of the above measures or if respiratory difficulty or a severe change in mental state occurs.

CITIES OVER 2000 METERS ABOVE SEA LEVEL

Addis Ababa, Ethiopia	2450m (8038 ft.)
Aspen, Colorado	2369m (7773 ft.)
Bogota, Colombia	2645m (8678 ft.)
Cajamarca, Peru	2640m (8662 ft.)
Cochabamba, Bolivia	2550m (8367 ft.)
Cuenca, Ecuador	2530m (8301 ft.)
Darjeeling, India	2265m (7431 ft.)

Guanajuato, Mexico	2500m (8202 ft.)
La Paz, Bolivia	3658m (12,001 ft.)
Laramie, Wyoming	2217m (7272 ft.)
Mexico, D.F. (Mexico City)	2308m (7572 ft.)
Pachuca, Mexico	2426m (7959 ft.)
Puebla, Pue., Mexico	2162m (7093 ft.)
San'a, Yemen Arab Republic	2377m (7800 ft.)
Simla, India	2202m (7224 ft.)
South Pole Station (USA), Antarctica	2800m (9186 ft.)
Toluca, Mexico	2680m (8793 ft.)
West Yellowstone, Montana, USA	2025m (6644 ft.)
Zacatecas, Mexico	2446m (8025 ft.)

ASTHMA

Exacerbation of asthma and other respiratory diseases may occur while traveling. Avoid smoke and other irritants to help prevent such attacks. Stress, excess exertion, cold air, and infection may also precipitate attacks. Use a cold-weather mask and precondition yourself before your trip if you are planning to exert yourself in a cold climate. Discuss your problems with your physician and ask for prescriptions for appropriate medications to take with you. Travel to high altitudes or cold climates and certain activities, such as scuba diving, may not be advisable for patients with respiratory problems. If any significant respiratory difficulties should arise while traveling, seek medical advice immediately.

AUTOMOBILE

Travel by auto can be safe and comfortable, although statistically it is the most dangerous form of travel. A good, safe driver and the use of seat belts are two major factors that contribute to a pleasant trip. Another factor is the size of the vehicle; generally, the larger the vehicle, the greater the comfort and safety.

Long periods of sitting in a car can aggravate lower back problems and varicose veins. Stop periodically to walk and stretch. People prone to swelling of the feet and lower legs should wear support hose and exercise their legs frequently. A rolled-up towel or jacket or a small pillow placed between the curved section of the lower back and the seat can help prevent and relieve lower back pain. Special pillows are available for this purpose.

For additional information see entries on *Driving* and *Motion Sickness*.

BABESIOSIS

Babesiosis is a parasitic disease found in very specific areas of Europe and the United States. In the United States, Babesiosis is endemic to the northeastern coastal regions. Infested areas include eastern Long Island and Fire Island in New York, and Nantucket Island in Massachusetts. The disease is transmitted by tick bite.

The signs and symptoms of babesiosis, which include intermittent fevers, enlarged spleen, and destruction of red blood cells, are similar to those of malaria. The parasite, babesia, is found in human red blood cells and even resembles certain forms of malaria under the microscope.

Some individuals who have been infected are well and show no signs of disease. Others may become ill as late as six weeks after contracting the parasites. Babesiosis can be fatal in patients whose spleens have been removed. Some patients with the disease have been cured with quinine and the antibiotic clindamycin.

BACK PROBLEMS

Most persons will suffer from backache sometime in their lives, and a significant portion will have relatively severe or recurrent backache. Handling back problems while traveling is no different from handling them at home. Unfortunately, lower back injury is not uncommon in travelers, especially those unaccustomed to carrying heavy luggage and sitting for long hours.

Avoid carrying more weight than you are used to. If you must carry luggage, be sure to do so properly, using your arms and legs while keeping your back straight, or invest in a set of "wheels," a folding luggage trolley. Get up periodically, at least hourly when awake, to walk and stretch. Avoid sleeping in abnormal positions or cramped spaces. If you have a known back problem, check with your doctor before traveling for advice and any prescription medication you may need to take with you.

Immediate relief from backache can sometimes be obtained by pressing the lower curved portion of your back against a firm flat surface, such as a wall or floor. Sit against the wall as if on an imaginary stool with your back pressed to the wall and your knees bent, or lie on the floor with your knees drawn up toward your stomach. Unfortunately, pain returns when the pressure ceases, but the temporary relief provided by this maneuver can sometimes help you to put on pants, shoes, and socks, tasks sometimes impossible when pain is severe. A back brace or tight wrap can often accomplish the same temporary relief but is usually less effective. Place a pillow or rolled-up blanket between your back and the seat to prevent or alleviate lower backache when you must sit for long periods.

If severe back pain with motion does occur while you are traveling, the best treatment is usually bed rest, an analgesic such as aspirin, massage, and cold or hot compresses. Consult a doctor for diagnosis and treatment.

Protect your back while traveling. Don't bend your back and lift heavy objects. Backache is second only to diarrhea as the spoiler of trips. Fortunately, most traveler's backaches subside with the passage of time. (See also *Automobile Travel*.)

BAROTRAUMA

Barotrauma refers to the discomfort and injury that can occur with rapid changes in air or water pressure. When rapid changes occur in the external air or water pressure, any entrapped body air undergoes a change in volume. This trapped gas expands with ascent and contracts, forming a partial vacuum, with descent. These volume changes place unusual stress on affected organs and tissues. This stress can result in pain or even rupture of soft tissue, such as the eardrum or lung tissue.

Descent in an airplane or while scuba diving can affect the ears, the sinuses, and the lungs. The most commonly involved area is the ear. Pressure changes result in inward bulging of the eardrum with resultant pain. This effect can be prevented by simple techniques that open the eustachian tube before descent. These maneuvers, which include yawning, Valsalva maneuver (taking a deep breath, holding it, and bearing down), and swallowing are described in the entry *Air Travel*. The relatively high water pressure encountered while diving can result in the accumulation of fluid in the middle ear (serous otitis media) or even rupture of the eardrum. In addition to the pain and loss of hearing that accompany rupture, dizziness (vertigo) and even vomiting may occur as cold water enters the middle ear. Vomiting under water can represent a major problem to a diver. Individuals with nasal congestion should not dive or fly, but anyone who must fly should take decongestants.

A more serious ear problem may occur in divers who perform a Valsalva maneuver while descending. Vertigo, tinnitus (noise in the ear) and deafness may result from rupture of the oval or round window in the middle ear. The development of any of these symptoms demands the attention of a physician.

Barosinusitis or sinus squeeze in divers refers to damage to the sinuses with pain and sometimes bleeding. Pain occurs over the sinuses, above, below or behind the eyes. This complication is less common than ear squeeze and is another reason why those with upper respiratory problems should not dive.

Divers who experience shortness of breath and bloody sputum may have lung squeeze. Lung squeeze is really a form of pulmonary edema (fluid in the lungs) resulting from pressure changes in the chest that can occur with deep, breath-holding dives. This uncommon problem requires sophisticated treatment with oxygen under pressure (PEEP). Patients with lung squeeze ought to be transported to a hospital as quickly as possible.

Ascent-related barotrauma occurs in divers who surface too quickly or who fly soon after diving. Trapped air expands and can stretch the organ involved or even cause rupture. When the gas is trapped and ruptures a portion of the lung, pneumothorax (collapsed lung) with chest pain and shortness of breath results. Air may rupture from the lung into the bloodstream and act as an embolus. These arterial gas embolisms can settle in vital organs such as the heart, lung or brain with resultant stroke, heart attack, seizure, or an episode of unconsciousness that occurs almost immediately (less than ten minutes) after surfacing. Divers can avoid these problems by letting out, not holding, breath while ascending and surfacing from a dive. Divers with chest pain, shortness of breath, unconsciousness, seizures, apparent stroke, or other serious difficulties should be immediately transported to a hospital. Hospital personnel must be informed to consider diving-related complications.

Another serious ascent-related problem is decompression sickness, or the bends. In this condition, nitrogen bubbles escaping into the blood, lymph and other tissues can cause problems in various body systems. Skin changes such as itching and mottling, although not serious, may indicate bends. Joint pain can be severe but is less serious than lung, heart, and brain involvement. Fatigue is present in almost all cases.

Nitrogen narcosis, or "rapture of the deep," is the euphoria and poor judgment resulting from nitrogen-gas effects on the brain. This form of intoxication, which occurs in scuba divers, can be avoided by using helium/oxygen mixtures instead of air which is 80% nitrogen.

Treatment for decompression sickness, nitrogen narcosis and arterial gas embolism requires a compression chamber. Emergency care facilities may have access to a compression chamber. If not, information can be obtained by calling DAN (Diving Accident Network) at 919-684-8111. Fast ground transport to the treatment center is preferred, where possible, but because speed is very important, victims must often be transported by helicopters flying below 1000 feet or planes with cabin pressure maintained at sea level.

BITES AND STINGS

BITES

Gila Monsters. The Gila monster is a nonagressive lizard found in the southwestern United States and Mexico. This animal is known to bite when teased or handled. Local tissue injury and systemic signs may persist for up to four days after the bite. Deaths have been reported within hours. No antivenin is available. The affected area should be cleansed, ice packs should be applied and medical care should be sought.

Snakes. Snake bites are relatively uncommon but can be serious. The bite of a poisonous snake constitutes a medical emergency and demands immediate care. The victim should be cautioned to rest and to keep the affected part still. Burning pain at the site of the bite, numbness, tingling of other body parts, swelling near the bite, and a general feeling of illness suggest a poisonous snake bite. Late complications of poisonous bites may include severe damage to the area involved, difficulty breathing, shock, and general toxicity. Cleanse snake bites with soap and water. The use of snake-bite kits or treatment by cutting the bite and sucking out blood are controversial and may result in infection if performed under nonsterile conditions.

An attempt should be made to identify the snake that caused the bite so that the proper antivenin can be administered. If the snake is dead, bring it with you to the emergency treatment facility. Do not, however, attempt to catch or transport a live snake.

The sooner professional treatment is started, the better the chances of survival. If no symptoms have occurred within thirty minutes after the bite, a poisonous bite is unlikely.

Nonpoisonous snake bites should be treated like other animal bites with local cleansing, prophylactic tetanus injections, and appropriate antibiotics, if necessary.

If you are traveling in an area where poisonous snakes may be encountered, it's best to be prepared. Obtain a book describing the snakes found in the area you intend to visit. Wear long pants and boots, and check your shoes and clothing before you put them on. Do not walk or reach into areas blindly. Be careful when exploring areas where snakes may hide, such as rotting logs, sunny rocks, and thick undergrowth. Carry a stick or other long object to probe questionable areas from a safe distance. If you are in a snake-infested area with no access to medical care, bring antivenin with you and know how to use it. Do not walk barefooted in snake-infested areas, especially at night or in areas where visibility is poor.

Spiders. Spider bites can be painful and dangerous. Do not let spider-bite victims exert themselves. Apply a cold pack or ice and seek medical assistance.

In the United States, most serious bites are inflicted by the brown recluse spider (fiddle shape on the abdomen and back) and the black widow spider (red hourglass on a black abdomen). The bite of the brown recluse spider results in severe local damage and occasionally causes kidney failure or systemic problems. The bite of the black widow spider is generally characterized by a brief sharp pain at the site of the bite, followed by cramping pain in the area within 25 to 60 minutes. The cramps may subsequently involve the entire body, especially the abdomen. The abdomen, however, is not tender to the touch. Other symptoms are nausea, vomiting, headache, sweating, drooling, twitching and numbness of the hands and feet. Symptoms usually improve after several hours but may subsequently return for a few days. Most patients recover after one week. Deaths have occurred, however, among small children and older adults. Occasionally, the bite goes unnoticed, and the abdominal pain is the most prominent symptom.

To treat a black widow spider bite bathe the area with warm water and transport the patient to a medical facility where more specific treatment, such as the administration of antivenin, intravenous calcium, pain killers, and local wound care can be rendered.

The bites of large, hairy spiders, such as tarantulas, cause only local damage in most instances. However, more generalized symptoms similar to those associated with black widow spider bites may occur. Cleanse such a bite with water and soap or an antiseptic, and apply ice.

Ticks. Ticks bite, cling to the flesh and suck the victim's blood until they are full and drop off. To remove an imbedded tick, grasp the tick body firmly using a handkerchief or a gauze pad and exert a gradually increasing pulling motion until the tick releases its hold. A drop of almost any liquid placed on the body of the tick facilitates removal. Try to ensure that all the tick's mouth parts are removed, and try not to kill the tick before it is removed. Parts left in the victim's body may result in infection or the growth of a nodule.

Certain ticks cause a type of paralysis called "tick paralysis." The victim will recover completely from this paralysis if the tick is removed.

Rocky Mountain spotted fever is an infectious disease found in various areas of the United States, especially the southeast, that is transmitted by certain ticks. Severe headache, fever, and rash are the signs and symptoms of this disease. The rash frequently begins on the arms and legs and subsequently spreads to the trunk. If untreated, Rocky Mountain spotted fever may be fatal. In some cases, there is no definite history of a tick bite. For this reason, a rash accompanied by a fever or a severe headache demands medical attention. Treatment consists of the administration of certain antibiotics, such as tetracycline or chloramphenicol. Sulfonamides should never be used.

For other illnesses caused by ticks, see entries on *Babesiosis*, *Lyme disease*, and *Colorado tick fever*.

Wild Animals. Animal bites frequently become infected. In addition, some bites carry the risk of serious disease, such as rabies. Cleanse all bites thoroughly with soap and water. Apply an antiseptic, such as Betadine, and an antibiotic cream such as Neosporin, and consult a doctor as soon as possible. If medical care will be delayed, take Keflex or another antibiotic.

Rabies is commonly caused by dog or cat bites in certain countries, such as India and Mexico, and in areas bordering these countries, like southern Texas. Pet and human rabies is rare in the United States and in many other countries, but some wild animals may carry rabies. For this reason, bites by bats, skunks, foxes, raccoons, ferrets, ground hogs, muskrats, and other wild animals must be treated by a physician as soon as possible.

INSECT BITES AND SKIN IRRITATIONS.

Insect bites may cause local reactions and may lead to infection. Such bites may also cause other diseases that may not become evident for varying periods after the bite. If an illness develops within weeks or months after traveling, tell your physician about your trip and mention any bites you may have received while traveling.

All insect bites should be thoroughly cleansed with soap and water. The application of ice may decrease the pain and itching associated with such bites.

Bedbug bites result in simple puncture wounds in nonallergic persons. Allergic individuals, however, may experience irritation or hives. Treatment consists of the administration of antihistamines.

Centipedes. Local skin irritation may result from centipede bites. Some tropical species, however, may cause pain, local skin damage, and generalized reactions, such as headache, dizziness, anxiety, and vomiting. Centipedes have one pair of legs per body segment, distinguishing them from millipedes, which have two pair per segment. Millipedes cannot inject venom, but some do spray a burning fluid in the eye and on the skin that may result in blistering. A millipede species found in Haiti can reportedly spray this fluid more than 30 inches.

Contact with caterpillars, cocoons, or wind-blown caterpillar fuzz can also result in skin irritation, specifically caterpillar urticaria (hives). The skin of persons afflicted with this condition may become red, irritated, and painful. Blisters or hives may develop immediately after contact. Tenderness and swelling of the local lymph nodes may also occur. The reaction usually subsides within 24 hours. Treatment consists of soaking the affected area and administering oral antihistamines. Pain killers may be given, if necessary.

Chiggers or redbugs are small mites that are found on foilage. Avoid contact with chiggers by using insect repellents and wearing protective clothing. A substance secreted by the chigger causes a small red bump that can be treated locally with calamine lotion. If itching is severe, an oral antihistamine may be taken.

Fleas. Flea bites result in tiny bumps that itch. These bumps are an allergic reaction to the flea's saliva and are usually found on the lower legs and the feet. Domestic pets and, in some cases, wild animals such as the prairie dog, are the usual sources of fleas. In some areas of the southwestern United States, fleas have been known to cause bubonic plague in humans, but normally the small itchy bumps are the only consequence of flea bites. These bumps may be treated with calamine lotion. To prevent flea bites, wear protective clothing, such as long pants and high socks. Flea-infested domestic pets should be treated to rid them of these pests.

Mosquitos. Malaria is a disease caused by parasites transmitted by the bites of infected mosquitoes (anopheles). The malaria parasites attack red blood cells. Most forms of malaria (but not *plasmodium falciparum*) also affect the liver. Periodic high fevers, chills, sweats, and headaches are the symptoms of malaria. In some forms of the illness, these symptoms may not become apparent until many months after leaving the infected area.

Sleeping under mosquito netting at night and staying in well-screened areas during mosquito feeding times (usually in the evening, but ask local residents) can decrease the chances of infection. Protective clothing should be worn and insect repellents should be used liberally on the clothes and body. The most effective repellents contain deet (N-N-diethyl-meta-toluomide).

Malaria is found in parts of Mexico, Haiti, Central America, South America, Africa, the Middle East, Turkey, India, China, Indonesia, and Oceania. Certain preventive measures are recommended by the U.S. Public Health Service to travelers planning to visit these areas. (See *Malaria*.)

Dengue is a viral disease, transmitted by day-flying mosquitoes, endemic to certain tropical and subtropical areas, including the Caribbean, Puerto Rico, St. Bartholomew, St. Martin, the Dominican Republic, Guadeloupe, St. Thomas, Curaçao, Brazil, Haiti, Jamaica, Oceania, the Philippines, Thailand, India, Africa, Israel, the Near East, Malaysia, Borneo, Hawaii, New Guinea, Japan, and Vietnam.

The symptoms of dengue usually appear within a week after the victim is bitten. Initial symptoms resemble those of a mild cold. Conjunctivitis may also be present. Later symptoms include severe headache, pain behind the eyes, backache, and leg pains. Eye movement pain, chills, fatigue, weakness, and changes in taste may also occur. The eyes frequently appear bloodshot, a rash may be present, and small lumps may be seen on the palate. Lymph nodes may enlarge. The illness usually resolves within one week, but a second bout accompanied by fever may subsequently occur. Some patients require many weeks to recover fully from the infection. Although no specific treatment exists for dengue, the disease is rarely fatal. The only methods of protection against dengue are avoiding mosquito bites by wearing protective clothing, staying indoors, and using insect repellent.

STINGS

Bees and Wasps. Stings by bees and wasps are rarely fatal unless the victim is allergic to these creatures, or is a child or a person of small build who receives a great many stings simultaneously.

A generalized reaction is characterized by difficulty breathing, generalized swelling, shock, and unconsciousness. Such a reaction is life-threatening and should be treated with cardiopulmonary resuscitation and an immediate injection of adrenaline. Anyone with a severe allergy to insects should discuss the advisability of desensitization with their physician and should carry adrenaline for self-administration. Caution should be exercised in areas where these insects are found. Protective clothing should be worn and perfumes and bright clothing should be avoided. Clothing and shoes should be checked before being put on.

Scorpions. Scorpion stings are painful but rarely fatal. A victim should be kept still, ice packs applied to the affected area, while medical assistance is sought. Some stings produce abnormal sensations, such as pins and needles and numbness at the site of the sting, that may spread to a larger area. In rare cases, generalized symptoms, such as nausea and vomiting, are produced, followed by coma or convulsions and, eventually, death caused by heart failure.

Sea Life. Contact with Pacific and other cone shells can lead to cone-shell poisoning, which causes pain, swelling, changes in the color of the skin and numbness at the site of the sting. Generalized symptoms such as lack of coordination, confusion, weakness and shortness of breath may also occur. Most victims recover within one day, but death has been known to occur within five hours of poisoning. General medical care and treatment of symptoms ought to be administered, and respiratory control may be required. Immediate medical care should be sought.

The fins, spines, tails and other poison-laden appendages of fish may also produce stings. Stings inflicted by dogfish, bullhead sharks, ratfish, scorpion fish, wenerfish, toadfish and catfish can cause pain and swelling. Hot compresses should be applied as soon as possible. Catfish stings may result in local tissue loss and require wound care and medical attention. Infections requiring antibiotic treatment may also occur. Generalized symptoms that develop may require appropriate medical treatment.

Jellyfish, Portuguese man-of-war, and similar creatures may inflict stings that cause symptoms ranging from burning and local discomfort to severe pain with redness and swelling. Abdominal cramps, muscle pain, weakness, nausea, shortness of breath and collapse may occur for up to one week after the sting. Deaths are rare. Treatment consists of the application of ammonia or some other alkaline substance and calamine, and the administration of analgesics and oral antihistamines. In severe cases, cortisone has been used.

Some **sea anemone** found in Mediterranean and African waters can cause stings resulting in a condition characterized by a rash and ulcers known as sponge diver's disease. In late summer and fall, victims develop more generalized symptoms such as chills, fever, nausea, headache, chills and occasionally complete collapse. Death has rarely occurred. Treatment is purely symptomatic.

Stings from the spines of the **sea urchin** result in painful local swelling and ulcers. Some victims develop weakness and paralysis of the face and tongue that lasts for several hours. Occasionally, death has occurred, usually as a result of drowning caused by the paralysis and shock.

Sponge poisoning can be caused when certain sponges are touched. This painful rash is treated by applying dilute acetic acid (vinegar). There are no long-term effects.

Stingray injuries occur frequently on the California coast. The bony tail of this creature causes an envenomized puncture wound or laceration. Part of the tail often remains in the wound. The affected area is painful and becomes red and swollen. Weakness and, less often, convulsions can occur and even death can result. The wound should be irrigated with large amounts of salt water, preferably hot, and then immersed in the hottest water that the victim can tolerate in order to destroy the venom. The patient should be taken to the hospital for definitive medical care, including removal of the fragments of the tail from the wound, tentanus prophylaxis, administration of antiserum, and treatment with antibiotics to prevent infection.

VENOMOUS ANIMAL LOCATIONS

Approximately 7,000 people in the United States receive snake bites each year. Most of these occur in the South, especially Texas. Snake bites usually result in fewer than twenty deaths per year in this country, while worldwide the annual total is about 40,000. Snake bites are much more common in tropical and subtropical countries than in temperate regions. Areas with a high snake-bite mortality include Burma, Brazil, India, and Bangladesh. Africa accounts for fewer than 1000 snake-bite deaths each year. Most deaths occur among natives of these particular countries. Venomous sea snakes are found in the Pacific and Indian oceans.

In addition to snakes, certain lizards, spiders, scorpions, insects and various sea creatures can inflict venomous bites or stings which can be quite painful and may become infected, but are rarely fatal. Stings by bees, wasps, hornets, and similar insects are serious only to those people allergic to the specific venom, unless multiple stings are inflicted, especially on small children. Ant bites result in similar problems. With the exception of insects and certain spiders, most of these poisonous creatures are found in warm tropical and subtropical areas of the world.

SNAKES

Asian pit vipers—*Asia*
Australian brown snakes—*Australia*
Black momba—*South and central Africa*
Boomslang—*African savannahs*
Cobra (common Asian)—*southern Asia*
Copperhead—*New England to Texas*
Coral snake—*southern U.S.*
Cottonmouth moccasin—*southern U.S., Virginia to Texas*
Death adder—*Australia*
Desert horned viper—*dry Africa and Western Asia*
European vipers—*Europe*
Fer-de-lance—*Martinique*
Gaboon viper—*south of Sahara*
King cobra—*southern Asia*
Kraits—*southern Asia*
Puff adder—*south of Sahara and Middle East*
Rattlesnake—*western hemisphere*
Ringhals or spitting cobra—*South Africa*
Russell's viper or Tic-Palonga—*Asia*
Saw-scaled or carpet viper—*dry areas India to Africa*
Sea snakes—*Pacific (except NE) and Indian oceans*
Sharp-nosed pit—*eastern China and Indochina*
Tiger snake—*Australia*
Yellow or cape cobra—*South Africa*
Yellowbeard—*Mexico to Brazil*

LIZARDS

Gila monster—*southwestern U.S. and Mexico*
Mexican beaded lizard—*Mexican west coast*

INSECTS

Ants, bees, wasps, hornets, etc.—*worldwide*

SPIDERS

Atrax—*Australia*
Black widow—*worldwide tropical and temperate*
Brown recluse or fiddleback—*all of U.S.*
Tarantulas—*worldwide*

SCORPIONS

Tropic and subtropical

SEA LIFE

Cone shells—*South Pacific, Indian oceans*
Octopus—*worldwide, especially warm waters*
Portuguese man-o-war—*warm water areas of world*
Sea wasps—*South Pacific*
Stingrays—*tropical and temperate seas, some fresh water*
Stonefish—*South Pacific, Indian oceans*

BLINDNESS

(See *Guide Dogs*)

BLOOD DISORDERS

Travelers with sickle cell anemia, sickle cell disease, or other severe anemias (indicated by a hemoglobin value below 8) may have some difficulty with air travel. The lower oxygen levels associated with airplane travel may result in inadequate oxygen to the tissues and could even result in an acute emergency, such as a "sickle cell crisis." Patients with these problems are advised against travel by air. If a heart or lung disease is also present, flying is contraindicated. (See *Air Travel*.)

BRUCELLOSIS

Brucellosis is basically a disease of domestic animals such as swine, cattle, goats, and sheep. It is transmitted to humans through the eating or drinking of contaminated milk products or by skin contact with infected animal tissue. In the United States, brucellosis is for the most part an occupational disease found primarily in slaughterhouse workers.

Travelers may contract brucellosis from milk, cheese or other dairy products made from unpasteurized milk, and from products made from the skins of infected animals. Nearly half of the cases in the United States can be traced to products originating in Mexico.

Countries reporting over 1000 cases of human brucellosis each year are Argentina, Greece, Iran, Italy, Mexico, Peru, and Spain.

Although the disease responds to antibiotics, it is often difficult to diagnose because of its nonspecific symptoms. Brucellosis is best prevented by avoiding milk, milk products and animal hides in developing countries.

CAMPING

Camping in the United States is relatively safe, but there are certain precautions recommended. You may no longer assume that clear, running water is safe to drink. All water should be treated by some method of purification. The simplest is to boil the water for ten minutes. Other simple techniques include the use of purification tablets, chlorination, or the addition of tincture of iodine. (See *Water* for a more complete description of these methods.)

Because insects are frequently an annoyance when camping, insect repellents and protective clothing are recommended.

The risk of contracting certain diseases is higher in campers because of the increased likelihood of contact with wild animals, which may carry rabies, tularemia, or plague, and insects which may transmit plague, Colorado tick fever, Rocky Mountain spotted fever, viral encephalitis, tularemia or tick paralysis. Insect-related illnesses are most commonly transmitted by mosquitoes, fleas and ticks. Rabbits (through handling of hides or butchering) and various biting animals account for most of the animal-transmitted diseases. Do not handle, tease, or approach wild animals. Avoid butchering and eating wild animals, especially rabbits. Wear rubber gloves when handling dead animals.

CHOLERA

Cholera is an infamous disease that can and has killed thousands during epidemics. Death is usually a result of dehydration and shock from the massive, watery bowel movements caused by a toxin that the cholera bacteria produces. This problem can now be treated successfully by aggressive oral replacement of fluids and the administration of sugar and electrolytes.

Prevention is simple: Avoid contaminated water. If you don't drink unsafe water, you cannot contract cholera. A vaccine is available, but it is not 100% effective. Some countries, however, require the cholera vaccine for entry.

See entries on *Water* and *Vaccines* for more information. Also, check the IAMAT country-by-country list for information concerning the safety of water in the areas you plan to visit. If you have any doubt about the safety of the water, don't drink it.

CIRCULATORY DISORDERS

(See *Heart Disease* and *Air Travel*.)

COLD WEATHER EXPOSURE

Proper dress and a reasonably good physical condition are essential for participation in outdoor activities during cold weather. The best way to dress depends not only on the activity, but also on the air temperature, the wind speed, and the humidity. In general, loose-fitting thermal underwear (both shirt and pants) provides the best base. Multiple layers of shirts and sweaters over this allows easy adjustments to changes in activity level or temperature since you can remove or replace a layer. Wear outer pants like jeans, two pairs of socks, and a relatively lightweight jacket that is resistant to both water and wind. Foot gear and mittens or gloves should be appropriate for the planned activities and should be water-resistant. Mittens are warmer than gloves. Head gear should cover the ears and head; a knitted cap is usually best.

For extremes of cold and wind, you may need a hooded parka, a face mask, and thermal boots. Before exposing yourself to below zero temperatures for periods of more than a few minutes, seek the advice of experienced local residents.

Shivering is the first sign of exposure to cold. As exposure continues, shivering ceases, and the body temperature drops lower and faster. Muscles become uncoordinated, then rigid and finally flaccid. If cooling continues, cardiac arrest will occur, usually at a body temperature of below 70°F (21° C). If the body temperature remains above 90° F (32° C), the patient should be kept dry and protected from the cold and wind. If

WIND CHILL FACTOR CHART

Estimated wind speed (in mph)	Actual Thermometer Reading (°F.)											
	50	40	30	20	10	0	-10	-20	-30	-40	-50	-60
	EQUIVALENT TEMPERATURE (°F.)											
calm	50	40	30	20	10	0	-10	-20	-30	-40	-50	-60
5	48	37	27	18	6	-5	-15	-26	-36	-47	-57	-68
10	40	28	16	4	-9	-24	-33	-46	-58	-70	-83	-95
15	36	22	9	-5	-18	-32	-45	-58	-72	-85	-99	-112
20	32	18	4	-10	-25	-39	-53	-67	-82	-96	-110	-124
25	30	16	0	-15	-29	-44	-59	-74	-88	-104	-118	-133
30	28	13	-2	-18	-33	-48	-63	-79	-94	-109	-125	-140
35	27	11	-4	-20	-35	-51	-67	-82	-98	-113	-129	-145
40	26	10	-6	-21	-37	-53	-69	-85	-100	-116	-132	-148
(Wind speeds greater than 40 mph have little additional effect.)	LITTLE DANGER (for properly clothed person). Maximum danger of false sense of security.				INCREASING DANGER Danger from freezing of exposed flesh.				GREAT DANGER			

the patient is awake and able to swallow, hot liquids should be given. When the body temperature falls below 90° F., immediate emergency care is required. Because some methods of rewarming can cause further injury and even death, the treatment of such patients should be undertaken only by experienced medical personnel.

Frostbite results when actual freezing of local tissues occurs. The toes, feet, fingers, hands, ears, and nose are the most commonly involved areas. The affected area initially feels cold, subsequently becomes painful, and finally numbs. At first, the area may appear pale or discolored and will be hard or firm. Later the color may change and swelling and blistering may occur. At this stage, the frostbite lesions may resemble a burn. Treatment consists of rewarming the frostbite area in hot water of 100 ° F (37.8 ° C). The area must not be allowed to refreeze after warming has occurred. Smoking will further compromise circulation to the affected part and should be avoided.

Wind can play a very important role in exposure to cold weather. The wind chill factor is a more accurate index than temperature of the effect of cold weather on the body. Winds up to 40 miles per hour cause an effect which is equivalent to a decrease in temperature; above 40 miles per hour, there is little additional effect. When you dress for cold weather activities, check the equivalent temperature on the chart below.

COLORADO TICK FEVER

Colorado tick fever is a viral illness passed to humans by the bite of an infected tick. In addition to Colorado, this disease is found in Idaho, Nevada, Wyoming, Montana, Utah, eastern Oregon, Washington, and California. The illness may be associated with fever, muscle pains, headache, eye pain, and light sensitivity. One clue to the diagnosis is a two-day period of high fever followed by a few days of weakness without fever and then a second phase of high fever lasting up to three days. Most patients recall a tick bite during the week before onset. Recovery is usually complete, although many individuals are generally weak for a variable period after the illness. (See *Ticks* under *Bites and Stings*.)

COMMON COLD

The so-called common cold is an infection of the nose and/or throat caused by a number of different viruses. Virtually everyone has experienced this upper-respiratory illness. The symptoms of nasal discharge, stuffiness, and fever usually last for three to seven days and spontaneously disappear. Illness persisting for more than one week suggests some other problem, such as a bacterial infection of the nose, throat, or sinuses or an allergy.

Decongestants, pain medication, such as Tylenol or aspirin, and vitamin C are frequently used in treating colds. If symptoms, especially fever, persist beyond one week or if a productive cough or a thick nasal or postnasal discharge develops, physicians often prescribe an antibiotic such as ampicillin, amoxicillin, erythromycin, or an oral cephalosporin. Anyone taking decongestants should read the label to be sure that they have none of the medical problems that could be made worse by the medication.

Favorite cold remedies vary. One is Drixoral, an over-the-counter medication, every 12 hours, plenty of fluids, 2 grams of vitamin C per day, and acetaminophen (Tylenol) for headache or other facial pain. If tenderness develops over the face or if a productive cough develops, I tend to prescribe 250 mg erythromycin four times daily.

High fever, generalized symptoms (such as muscle aches and chills), deep cough, and symptoms other than those of the nose or throat suggest some problem more serious than a cold. In such cases consult a physician.

DEAFNESS

Individuals who are completely or partially deaf can usually travel with only a little more difficulty than those who hear well. When traveling by commercial carrier, identify yourself to the attendant so that auditory messages, such as safety procedures on airplanes or train station stops, can be provided for you. Hearing guide dogs are of great benefit to hearing-impaired travelers. If you have a hearing guide dog, read *Guide Dogs* entry.

DIABETES

Almost all diabetics may travel safely, but the illness must be taken seriously and certain preparations must be made to ensure a safe and comfortable trip. Before a trip is considered, diabetes should be reasonably well-controlled and the diabetic patient should understand the prescribed diet and medication. If any special problems are associated with the disease, such as a poor sensation in the feet or poor eyesight, special precautions should be taken. Most important is a knowledge of how to monitor blood and urinary glucose, how to diagnose excessively high or low blood sugar, and how to alter medication and food intake to compensate for excessive glucose levels. A diabetic patient who does not feel confident in his or her ability to control the disease is not ready for any significant travel unless accompanied by a nurse or other companion who is able and willing to assume responsibility for control of the patient's disease.

The diabetic patient should visit a physician before any major trip. The physician can provide advice and prescribe medication that will be needed. Items essential for the trip include a full supply of any medications taken regularly, extra prescriptions in case the medication is lost, disposable syringes for insulin users, tapes for testing urinary and blood glucose, along with instructions for their use, and a letter on the physician's stationery identifying the patient as a diabetic.

The diabetic patient should wear a Medic Alert bracelet or necklace, and carry an identification card, indicating that he or she is a diabetic. If travel to a foreign country is planned, the identification card should be in the language of that country, if possible. A fast-acting source of carbohydrates, such as candy or sugar cubes, as well as a more slowly absorbed source of sugar, such as crackers with peanut butter or cheese, should also be carried.

Any drastic changes in diet should be avoided. The airlines will provide a special meal for diabetic patients if notified 24 hours before flight time. Patients who are more active while traveling and especially those who will participate in athletic activities to which they are not accustomed will find that increasing their usual insulin dosage (by approximately 20%) and consuming additional carbohydrates during strenuous physical activity will help. When traveling across time zones by air, the diabetic patient should not reset his or her watch until settled at the destination. In this way, timing of meals and medication will be facilitated. Urine should be monitored at least daily while traveling, even if this is not normally done at home. If traveling alone, the diabetic patient should inform appropriate persons, such as flight attendants, that he or she is diabetic so that help can be provided if hypoglycemia should occur.

The crises that can occur in diabetic patients may present major problems while traveling. The most dangerous of these is a severe hypoglycemic reaction that may lead to unconsciousness or seizures. For this reason, it is better to err on the side of a little less strict control of diabetes while traveling. Hypoglycemia should be avoided and a fast-acting form of sugar should be carried.

Because hyperglycemia or even diabetic acidosis takes longer to develop than low blood sugar, elevated blood sugar is less of a threat during travel. Hyperglycemia should almost never occur if glucose is monitored regularly and properly. However, an acute illness may result in elevations of blood sugar, even if the patient is not eating. Nausea and vomiting or diarrhea can result in excessive blood sugar or a very low blood sugar. All prophylactic measures should be taken to prevent and treat acute illnesses (see *Diarrhea*, and *Emergencies*, *Vomiting*). Blood sugar should be monitored frequently during any illness.

The diabetic patient should obtain a list of available doctors in every area he or she will visit. These local doctors will be able to replace lost medication, identify insulin in foreign countries (see accompanying table), or assist with diabetic control.

A publication entitled *Vacationing With Diabetes, Not From Diabetes* is available from the E.R. Squibb Pharmaceutical Company, Lawrenceville-Princeton Road, Princeton, NJ 08540.

RECOMMENDATIONS FOR DIABETICS

Insulin users

- Take regular insulin with you even if you don't ordinarily use it.
- Disposable syringes may be used more than once.
- Take enough insulin for the entire trip.
- If you obtain insulin in a foreign country, consider that it differs in potency and make the appropriate adjustments (U-80 Insulin, all pork).
- Check urine at least daily.
- Accept a slightly higher blood glucose value than you feel represents good control at home.

- Wear identification.
- Carry a card or letter from your doctor outlining diagnosis, medications, and need for needles (in the appropriate foreign language).

All diabetics

- Visit your doctor before your trip, get prescriptions and a checkup.
- Carry test tapes for blood and urine glucose; monitor daily.
- Understand and control your own disease.
- Carry a supply of all necessary medications.
- Wear diabetic identification (bracelet or necklace plus card).
- Have names of doctors in area you will visit.
- Take more carbohydrates (50%) when exercising vigorously.

NAMES OF DIABETIC MEDICATIONS IN FOREIGN COUNTRIES

U.S. Name	*Foreign Names*
Acetohexamide (Dymelor)	Dimelin, Ordinel
Chlorpropramide (Diabinese)	Catanil, Chloronase, Chlorodiabet, Diabetoral, Millinese
Tolazamide (Tolinase)	Orabetta, Tolisan, Norgylcin
Tolbutamide (Orinase)	Rastinon, Artosin, Dolital, Diabin, Mellitus D, Yosulant Oralin, Orsinin
Insulin (regular)	Actrapid
Insulin, NPH	Monotard, Lentard
Not available in U.S.	Daonil, Eugleucon, Daolin

DIARRHEA, TRAVELER'S

Traveler's diarrhea is a term used to describe any form of diarrhea that occurs while traveling. This condition is frequently caused by certain bacteria such as *Escherichia coli*, shigella, or salmonella, but may also be caused by viruses or parasites, such as amoeba or *Giardia*. These various pathogens are ingested with contaminated food or drink.

Avoiding infected food and water is the best approach to the prevention of traveler's diarrhea. Developing nations and tropical countries are the areas of greatest risk but some travelers to so-called developed countries may also develop diarrhea. Eat only cooked, hot food and drink only sealed sterile beverages, such as beer and carbonated beverages. Avoid water and ice completely, as well as fresh fruits and vegetables in Mexico, Central America, South America, parts of Europe, and the Orient. Certain hidden sources of infection include glasses washed in contaminated water and water used when brushing the teeth. Water can be purified by boiling or by using chlorine or water purification tablets.

Certain prophylactic medications may be useful in preventing diarrhea (discuss the advisability of taking these with your physician):

Doxycycline—The recommended dose of this prescription drug is 200 mg on the first day of travel and 100 mg daily thereafter. Side effects may include nausea, vaginitis, sunburn, and, later, diarrhea. Children younger than nine years of age should not receive doxycycline.

Pepto-Bismol liquid—The effective dose of this over-the-counter drug is 60 ml (2 oz.) four times daily. There is no proof that Pepto-Bismol tablets or smaller doses of the liquid are effective. Use of this drug may cause the stool to turn black.

Trimethoprim-Sulfamethoxazole—One double-strength tablet (DS) of this prescription drug daily is recommended for the prevention of diarrhea.

Water combined with juices, some form of sugar, salt and baking soda may be used to replace fluids and other materials in individuals who have become dehydrated as a result of diarrhea. One recommended combination for replacing potassium, sugar, and salt is eight ounces of fruit juice, one-half teaspoon of honey or corn syrup, and a pinch of regular table salt.

Another mixture for replacing bicarbonate and fluids is eight ounces of boiled or carbonated water and one-fourth teaspoon of baking soda. These two different mixtures should be drunk alternately and supplemented with carbonated beverages. Solid food, milk, caffeine, and alcohol should be avoided until recovery is apparent.

DISABLED PERSONS

Disabled persons can and do travel. Individuals who are active and functioning within their own community are able to travel. Those who are disabled can educate themselves concerning their specific physical limitations and those resources available to compensate for these restrictions. Functional level is often determined more by personal drive and determination than by any specific physical defect.

A visit to the physician for a checkup and advice before traveling is essential. Physical therapists can also provide helpful and practical advice regarding physical disabilities. Airlines, bus companies, and travel agencies, as well as most service and entertainment facilities, will provide special assistance if they are made aware of special needs. Airlines will transport disabled persons from gate to gate, provide wheelchairs and oxygen, and allow advance boarding of a flight. When reservations are made, arrangements for special needs should be discussed. Reservations ought to be made well in advance and disabled persons need to check in as early as possible.

More preparation and planning are necessary if disabled persons want to travel off the beaten path. The further you go from cities, towns and the usually traveled routes, the less likely you are to find special accommodations for the disabled. In order to travel safely and in relative comfort in out-of-the-way areas, disabled persons must be relatively self-sufficient.

There are a number of good publications available to help anyone who is planning to travel while disabled:

- *Access Travel: Airports—A Guide to Accessibility of Terminals.* Free. Access America, Washington, DC 20202.
- *Consumer Information About Air Travel for the Handicapped.* Free. TWA.

- *Access AMTRAK, National railway passenger corporation,* Office of Customer Relations, Amtrak, P.O. Box 2709, Washington, DC 20013.
- *The Wheelchair Traveler.* c/o Douglas Annard, Ball Hill Road, Milford, NH 03055.
- *Access to the World: A Travel Guide for the Handicapped,* by Louise Weiss. Facts on File, 460 Park Ave. S., New York, NY 10016.

DIVING EMERGENCIES

Scuba diving accidents are often avoidable. Do not dive without proper instruction and equipment and never dive alone. Alcohol is a major risk factor to divers; never dive when you have been drinking. Drowning is the most frequent cause of deaths associated with diving. Other common causes of death in divers are an exhausted air supply, panic, fatigue, and equipment failure. Hypothermia, toxic plants, dangerous sea creatures, and physical injury constitute other dangers to divers. Proper training and strict adherence to safe diving rules are critical in preventing emergencies associated with diving.

Decompression sickness or the "bends" is a serious condition that may develop during or after a dive. Joint pain, with or without itching and rash, occuring within the first 24 hours after a dive must be considered a symptom of decompression sickness until proven otherwise. Other symptoms may include fatigue, headache, abdominal pain, chest pain, dizziness, nausea, vomiting, backache, weakness, a speech disorder, breathlessness, and urinary difficulties. The treatment for decompression illness consists of recompression in a hyperbaric chamber as soon as possible and requires transport of the patient to an emergency facility. Special consultation can be obtained by contacting the United States Air Force, School of Aerospace Medicine, in San Antonio, Texas, at 512-536-3281 during the day or 512-536-3278 at night.

Shallow-water blackout is another potential danger associated with diving. This form of unconsciousness occurs when divers who are not using scuba gear hyperventilate before holding their breath.

Unconsciousness while diving is disastrous and will result in drowning. Oxygen, nitrogen, carbon monoxide or carbon dioxide toxicity can cause unconsciousness in divers using scuba gear. Running out of air will result in blackout as well. Near drowning or hyperventilation are the two most common causes. Most of these situations are preventable through training and meticulous attention to techniques. However, even the most cautious diver may experience accidents. For that reason, always dive with at least one other reliable person.

Anything out of the ordinary, like apprehension, air hunger and euphoria, twitching, light-headedness, ringing ears, nausea, or weakness, should alert you that something may be wrong. Pay attention to these symptoms and if they occur, discontinue your dive and signal for help before more serious symptoms arise.

The following medical conditions usually temporarily disqualify an individual from diving:

upper respiratory infection

bronchitis

perforated eardrum

severe respiratory allergies

pregnancy

nasal obstruction.

Many medical authorities believe that persons with the following medical problems should never dive:

seizure disorder

diabetes requiring insulin

alcoholic or drug abuse

severe anemia

recent head trauma

coronary artery disorder

emphysema

lung disorders.

If you are considering diving and have any medical problem, discuss the situation with your doctor first. Asthma, previous pneumothorax, migraine, previous middle ear surgery, hypertension, visual problems, and previous barotrauma of any kind dictate a trip to your physician for an examination and final discussion about the advisability of diving.

DOCTORS (LOCATING A PHYSICIAN)

Locating a physician while traveling may not be easy, especially in foreign countries or areas away from the usual tourist routes. The quality of medical care varies greatly throughout the world, and the high level of care that most Americans are accustomed to is not always available.

Individuals with a significant medical problem should ask their own physicians for the names of doctors in the areas that they plan to visit. If the physician cannot furnish any names, friends, relatives, and business associates from the areas to be visited can often be helpful. If an individual with no specific referrals should become ill while traveling in the United States, the best choice is usually to report to an emergency room. The standards of emergency room care are now fairly uniform throughout the United States. Hotels often have physicians on call who will see guests in their rooms; the hotel telephone operator or front desk can help in contacting the house physician. However, variations in the quality of care available from hotel physicians are even greater than those found among emergency room physicians. For the seriously ill traveler, the emergency room is the best choice.

Excellent medical care is usually available at the infirmaries of major U.S. international airports. Simply ask at any of the airline counters for directions to the infirmary. In addition to emergency medical care, the infirmary personnel can provide other important up-to-date health information related to travel.

Major sports arenas and race tracks usually have a first-aid station or infirmary that can provide emergency care. The quality of care varies greatly at these stations, but the immediate availability can be convenient and even life saving. Most employees of such facilities will be able to provide directions to the medical care area.

Foreign travel is a completely different situation. Some countries, such as Canada and the United Kingdom, provide good medical care by English-speaking physicians at a reasonable charge or even at no cost. In other countries, you must be prepared to handle your own medical problems or, when possible, to travel to an area where good care is available.

The best source of physicians, hospitals and health-care facilities outside the United States is a booklet published by IAMAT, the International Association for Medical Assistance to Travellers (see *IAMAT*). The directory (which is reprinted in the back of this book) and membership in IAMAT is free from IAMAT, 736 Center Street, Lewiston, NY 14092. Updated annually, the directory lists facilities, telephone numbers, and set fees. By obtaining an IAMAT membership identification card you are guaranteed qualified medical care by English-speaking physicians on a twenty-four-hour basis. I recommend that anyone who travels outside of the United States join IAMAT and carry their directory. Donations of any amount are suggested to support IAMAT, which exists solely on voluntary contributions. Donations are tax deductible.

Another list of doctors abroad is available from Intermedic, 777 Third Avenue, New York NY 10017, telephone 212-486-8974.

If you are unable to find a physician, call the local hospital or visit the emergency room in English-speaking countries. In other countries call the American embassy or consulate and ask if they will provide you with physician names and telephone numbers.

It is usually advisable to deal with your medical problems at your location. In the event that you must return home, travel by commercial airlines, if possible. Some carriers will make special arrangements if you must travel by stretcher. In some cases, the U.S. State Department has helped make special arrangements on commercial or military flights, but the cost for these arrangements can be astronomical.

Some companies specialize in emergency assistance to member travelers at a reasonable rate. These include:

International SOS Assistance
2 Neshaminy Interplex
Trevose, PA 19047 (215-244-1050)

This company will refer you to physicians who speak English, pay transportation to the nearest medical facility, offer an interest-free loan for medical bills, relay your medical history from home, and offer other services. You may obtain annual, monthly, or weekly membership.

Assist-Card
745 Fifth Avenue
New York, NY 10022 (800-221-4564)

Assist-Card will provide English-speaking doctors, pay up to $300 of medical bills, and transport you to the nearest medical facility or arrange for your return home (and pay for the trip if it is judged medically necessary). There is a daily fee for coverage.

Near, Inc.
1900 N. MacArthur Blvd.
Oklahoma City, OK 73127 (800-654-6700)

Near, Inc. offers a 24-hour toll-free hotline for travelers and their families at home. This hotline may be used to contact family members for emergencies or to arrange an emergency trip home. If you can travel only by stretcher, Near pays the full cost of transportation. A traveler may also obtain foreign hospital insurance coverage. You may purchase a monthly membership.

DRIVING

Driving is one of the most frequent means of travel, but it is also one of the most dangerous. With a little planning and adherence to some simple rules, however, you can decrease this danger considerably.

Certain illnesses tend to increase the risk of an automobile accident, especially when these illnesses are poorly controlled. In patients with diabetes, epilepsy, cerebrovascular disease, heart disease, chronic lung disease, depression, hypertension, arthritis, peripheral vascular disease, or kidney disease, the illness should be under good control for some period of time before driving is attempted. Individuals with poor vision or blindness in one eye and those who are deaf should be cautious when driving, especially in areas unfamiliar to them. Anyone who is senile or has suffered a recent severe physical defect should not drive.

Larger cars are safer than smaller cars, and very small cars, sports cars, and motorcycles are the least safe vehicles. Seat belts should always be used when traveling.

Before a trip, have your vehicle checked and in good, safe running condition. Learn what to do if emergency situations occur while driving. If your accelerator becomes stuck, put the car in neutral and come to a stop at the side of the road while you are attempting to free the accelerator with your foot.

If the brakes fail, pump them and gradually apply the emergency brake. If these maneuvers do not stop the car, shift into a lower gear to slow the car and steer uphill, if possible. When these methods are unsuccessful in stopping the car, and impact is imminent, direct the car toward an object, such as a hedge, that will gradually slow you down, rather than toward an immovable barrier.

When steering fails, gradually brake the car and simultaneously warn others by blowing the horn and turning on the headlights and emergency flashers.

If a blowout occurs in a front tire, remove your foot from the accelerator and turn the wheel to the side opposite the blowout. Gradually brake the car and steer off the road.

Fire in the engine may constitute a great danger. In the event of such a fire, pull safely off the road and quickly evacuate the car. If the fire is very small, you may try to put it out with a fire extinguisher, but if it is not easily controlled, get far away from the car. Call the nearest fire department and the police.

A dropped drive shaft is indicated by rumbling vibrations under the car, accompanied by a loss of rear-wheel drive and the possible loss of control as the shaft drags on the roadway. Slow the car gradually, but don't steer off the road until you have nearly stopped. This maneuver will prevent the shaft from digging into the soft shoulder and flipping the car.

During the seconds before an impending crash, press your head against the headrest or seat back. Lift your feet off the floor, fold your arms across your abdomen, and grasp your elbows to minimize injury. Your seatbelt and harness should be on.

Car sickness may be avoided or minimized by sitting in the front seat, driving, focusing on distant objects, and keeping the car windows open. The prophylactic use of antihistamines before travel may also help. However, because these drugs may decrease alertness, they should not be used by the driver.

If an accident should occur, try to remain calm. If the car is on fire or is sinking in water, get out as fast as possible through an open window or door. Avoid cutting yourself on jagged metal or broken glass. After an accident, take a few minutes to feel your head, neck, abdomen, chest, and extremities to check for injuries. Determine whether or not you can move your arms and legs. Cautiously get out of the car and check to determine if your legs will bear your weight. Stop any bleeding with direct pressure. Assist anyone else who is injured and perform cardiopulmonary resuscitation (CPR) and first aid as needed. Remember that anyone who is unconscious may have a neck as well as a head injury; do not bend the neck if there is any possibility of neck injury. Obtain emergency help as soon as possible.

DROWNING, NEAR

Victims of near drowning require immediate attention. If no spontaneous breathing is apparent or no pulse can be felt, cardiopulmonary resuscitation (CPR) should be performed. CPR should be continued until spontaneous breathing and the pulse have returned.

Some patients will recover from a near drowning with no permanent damage, even after being submerged for long periods of time. This is especially true for children who have undergone lengthy submersion in cold water. All victims of near drowning, however, should be referred for medical examination. Some who appear to be well will develop respiratory symptoms over the next twenty-four hours. All those who have experienced a near drowning should be seen by a physician.

DRUG ABUSE

All forms of drug abuse are dangerous to your mental and physical health. When traveling, there is the added danger of very serious legal difficulties and very severe penalties for even minor offenses, not to mention the unpredictability and dangerous contents of the drugs themselves in foreign countries.

If you should encounter someone who seems to be having a drug-related problem, try to keep them calm and get them to a medical facility. Make an attempt to find out what drug they have ingested, how much, and when they took the last dose.

EMERGENCIES

Illness or injury that occurs while traveling can usually be dealt with if you are mentally and physically prepared before your trip. Your compact traveler's medical kit (see p. 5) should be checked and updated before each trip. Show the list of its contents to your physician for comments and recommendations concerning your own unique medical needs. Once you decide on the specific items you need to carry while traveling, keep a list with your travel kit and check it before each trip.

A book on first aid should be part of any traveler's baggage. Many such books are available, and you should become familiar with them before traveling. One simple but rather complete book is *The AMA Handbook of First Aid and Emergency Care* published by Random House. Check the various first-aid books in your library and book stores, choose one, and use it at home so that you become familiar with it before your trip. Most emergencies you will encounter will be covered in this valuable resource.

ABDOMINAL PAIN

Abdominal pain may indicate a minor upset related to overindulgence in food or drink, a self-limited bowel disease, or a serious and even life-threatening disorder. Three factors should be considered when attempting to identify the cause of such pain. The first is the severity of the pain. The more severe the pain, the greater the likelihood that it represents serious disease. The second factor, the location of the pain, will aid in determining possible specific illnesses. The speed of onset is the third factor. Pain that is gradual in onset often signifies a medical disorder, whereas a very sudden onset pattern suggests some type of physical obstruction or perforation.

When pain is mild, poorly localized, and gradual in onset, simple remedies, such as a hot bath, a bowel movement, or the use of mild analgesics, such as Tylenol, may be tried. An antacid will sometimes help in relieving upper abdominal, dyspepsic-type pain. Avoid enemas, laxatives, or strong analgesics. If pain persists for more than one hour, is severe, or sudden in onset, take nothing orally and seek medical help. This same approach should be followed in cases in which the pain is mild but the patient appears to be seriously ill. Upper abdominal pain can sometimes be caused by heart disease (see following section on chest pain).

CHEST PAIN

Physicians consider chest pain a medical emergency until certain diagnoses are ruled out. Heart attacks, blood clots to the lung, collapsed lung, and pneumonia are a few of the more serious problems that may cause chest pain.

Generally, the younger a person is the greater the likelihood the chest pain is of a nonserious nature. However, no age is immune to serious chest problems, and anyone with this symptom should see a doctor.

Certain associated symptoms, such as shortness of breath, sweating, fever, or collapse, suggest that the pain is of an urgent character. When chest pain is associated with pain or aching in the neck, jaw, shoulders or arms, heart disease is a likely possibility. Palpitations, sweating, nausea, collapse, fainting, or an irregular pulse also suggest a heart problem and make an immediate examination by a physician mandatory. Shortness of breath and worsening of the pain with breathing suggest a pulmonary embolism (clot to the lung), pneumothorax (collapsed lung), or pneumonia. These are all life-threatening conditions and demand immediate medical treatment.

There is no safe, effective first aid for chest pain. Keep the patient quiet, administer oxygen if available, and transport the person to a hospital as soon as possible.

CHOKING

Choking usually indicates blockage of the airway by some foreign body, such as food or mucus. A choking victim's ability to cough forcefully or to speak indicates only partial obstruction. Such patients should be encouraged to cough, but no further action should be taken. Any maneuvers attempted could lead to complete obstruction.

If it is known that the victim is choking on something swallowed but can cough, speak, or breathe, simply call for help.

If this victim cannot cough, speak, or breathe, a chest thrust of some type should be performed:

- Grasp the patient from behind in a quick firm bear hug if he or she is sitting or standing.
- If on the floor, roll the victim onto his or her back; place the heel of one hand in the center of the chest, place the other hand over it and press down four times.
- If unsuccessful, tilt the head back, open the mouth and remove any objects with a sweep of your index finger.
- If still unsuccessful, give the patient four firm back blows and repeat one of the chest maneuvers described above.
- Keep checking the mouth and applying chest thrusts and back blows until successful.

- If after two minutes you are not successful, try CPR.

Taking a course in CPR will allow you to learn and practice these life-saving maneuvers.

CONVULSIONS

Although frightening to the observer, convulsions may be easily handled. The basic goal of emergency care is to prevent the patient from choking on his or her own tongue, dentures, or secretions and to avoid injury from a fall or violent motions. Try to break any falls by easing the patient down, move dangerous objects out of the way, and place a soft object, such as a towel or newspaper, between the patient's teeth to prevent tongue biting. Do not try to hold the victim down or use force to restrain.

During the convulsion, the patient may not breathe, but no attempt should be made, then, at resuscitation. After the seizure, cardiopulmonary resuscitation (CPR) may be performed if necessary. When the seizure has ended, let the patient rest. Turn his or her head to the side or place the patient abdomen-down in order to prevent inhalation of vomit or secretions. Check for any indication of a medical illness associated with seizures (such as a card in the patient's wallet or a medical alert bracelet, necklace, or tag). Epilepsy, diabetes, a high fever (especially in children), alcoholism, brain disease, head injury, and certain drugs may be associated with seizures.

The victim of a seizure should always be seen by a physician. After a seizure, the patient is often confused and uncooperative and may resist or refuse medical care. Emergency transportation should be arranged, if necessary.

CPR INSTRUCTIONS

If the person is conscious and able to talk, no CPR is necessary.

If the person is breathing normally, no CPR is necessary.

If the patient is unconscious and not breathing normally:

- Call for help (loudly, without leaving the patient).
- Place the patient flat on his or her back, strip clothes off chest.

- Kneel by the patient's side and pinch the nose closed.
- Lift the chin with your other hand to bend the head back.
- Cover the patient's mouth with yours.
- Force four deep breaths of air into the lungs as if you were blowing up a balloon.

Recheck the patient; if he or she is moving or breathing normally, discontinue CPR; if not:

- Place the heel of your hand on the center of his or her chest right between the breasts.
- Place the other hand on top of that hand and push down on the heels of your hand 1 to 2 inches. Repeat this motion 15 times as if you were pumping the chest.
- Pinch the nose, lift the chin as before, and administer four more deep breaths.
- Pump the chest 15 times as before.
- Keep repeating this cycle until help is available.
- Stop only when the patient appears to be moving or breathing normally.

DENTAL PROBLEMS

Dental problems while traveling may usually be avoided by visiting your dentist periodically, especially before leaving on an extended vacation. If, while traveling, a permanent tooth is dislodged, it should be replaced in the gum immediately and held in place while emergency care is sought. Any delay in replacing the tooth will decrease the chances of its survival. If a tooth is loosened or pushed out of alignment, reposition it immediately and hold it in place until the dentist can be seen. Any break or fracture of a tooth requires dental care. Toothaches may be treated with analgesics, such as aspirin, but such treatment is only a temporary measure. Any swelling, fever, or severe pain signifies a more serious problem and requires attention as soon as possible. If you are in an area where it is impossible to obtain dental care, consider taking an antibiotic and washing your mouth frequently with warm salt water. You may be able to contact an English-speaking dentist with the help of IAMAT-listed physicians (see *IAMAT*).

DIZZINESS

Dizziness is a nonspecific term frequently used to describe a light-headed or giddy feeling. This symptom can signify serious underlying disease although it is usually an indication of a less serious condition. If you are dizzy, driving or performing tasks that require full attention and coordination should be avoided. Check for fever, a rapid heat beat, or signs of acute illness. If you suspect your blood pressure has decreased with standing or sitting, keep supine and have someone seek medical care. Vertigo or a feeling of spinning can indicate problems within the nervous system and requires medical attention. While someone seeks medical care, stay quiet and still. Do not smoke or take medications, alcohol, or drugs.

FEVER

Fever usually indicates some type of infection, although fever may also be caused by many other medical problems, such as allergic reactions and tumors. Although acetaminophen (such as Tylenol), aspirin, and other antipyretics can decrease some fevers, use of such drugs is controversial. There is usually no urgent need to lower the temperature in patients with fevers of less than 105° F. except with children who may experience febrile seizures. Every effort should be made to identify the cause of fever, and the patient should ingest fluids in order to avoid dehydration. Fevers that occur after returning from a trip may be an indication of a disease contracted while traveling. Be sure to tell your physician of your travels so that consideration can be given to all possible causes.

HEADACHE

Headache is one of the most common human afflictions. Mild headaches are often not serious and may be treated with rest, massage, cold compresses, and mild analgesics. Certain headaches, however, indicate a serious underlying illness and require expert medical care. New, severe, and increasing headaches may be serious. Difficulty with vision, fever, a stiff neck, mental changes, vomiting, or loss of muscle function are signs of serious disorders and demand prompt professional attention.

ITCHING

Itching is frequently caused by a rashes (see *Rashes* below for further information). When itching occurs without a rash, the possible causes include allergies, liver disease, or irritation by clothing, plants, or other materials in contact with the skin. Scratching will usually aggravate itching and should be avoided. The involved areas should be bathed in cool water, and calamine lotion should be applied. For severe itching, an antihistamine (e.g., Vistaril) may be useful. Persistent itching may indicate infection with parasites (e.g., fleas, scabies, lice) and a physician should be consulted.

LUMPS AND BUMPS

Lumps and bumps on the skin or under the skin may be reactions to insect or parasite bites, or may indicate allergic or infectious disease. Occasionally they may represent tumors. Any persistent lump should be checked by a physician. Do not attempt to probe a lump with sharp objects, such as needles. If the mass is red and/or tender, it may represent a local infection that will respond to warm water soaks and antibiotics (e.g., Keflex). Such infections should be treated by a physician.

RASHES

Rashes are common medical problems that are often transient and frequently resolve without treatment. The diagnosis of a rash can be difficult and depends on the character of the lesions, their distribution, the presence of itching and any associated signs and symptoms. Never scratch a rash. Approaches to the symptomatic treatment of rashes are outlined in the preceding section on itching.

Rashes commonly occur at home as well as abroad. If a rash appears while traveling, the problem is likely to be a common one rather than some unusual exotic disease contracted during your trip. However, when you do seek medical attention, be sure to inform your physician of your travels, as well as any medication or immunizations you have received.

A rash accompanied by a fever is more likely to be a sign of an infectious disease, whereas rashes that itch tend to be allergic reactions. If severe illness occurs along with a rash, the problem may be serious, and medical care should be sought.

An individual who develops a rash should discontinue any medication that is not essential. In the absence of illness and fever, there is usually no urgent need to be examined. Calamine lotion may be applied to the areas that itch. An antihistamine, such as Dramamine or Vistaril, may relieve itching that doesn't respond to calamine. A physician should be consulted if the rash persists or becomes worse, or if other symptoms such as headache, diarrhea, chills, fever, stiff neck, sore throat, joint pain, or difficulty with breathing are present.

If a rash appears on an area of the skin that is in contact with jewelry, clothing, or some other object, removing the material from contact with the skin may result in the healing of the "contact dermatitis." Over-the-counter hydrocortisone-containing creams may help in some cases of rash, but may worsen others, such as infections and ringworm.

SPRAINS

Overstretching of the ligaments and fibers of a joint can result in sprains. Sudden and forceful movements, such as twisting an ankle, are the usual causes of sprains. The symptoms can vary from little or no pain and swelling in cases of mild stretching, to tearing with marked pain and swelling. The area may be tender to the touch and more painful with movement. These findings are also present when certain bones are broken (fractures), as well as with severe sprains. Radiographic examination is the only way to rule out a possible fracture.

Treatment of sprains consists of applying cold compresses and elevating the injured area. An elastic bandage may be used to hold a cold compress in place. Cold compresses should be replaced after approximately twenty minutes. Because the bandage will tighten as swelling occurs, it should be checked frequently. The veins at some distance from the bandage should not stand out or bulge, and pulses should be easily felt. Distended veins, an absent pulse, cold, numbness, or swelling away from the bandage may indicate an excessively tight bandage that should be removed. If pulses are still not present, vessel injury should be suspected and medical care should be sought immediately. If pain occurs with use of the injured part, movement should be avoided.

ULTRAVIOLET EYE INJURY

Ultraviolet eye injury (UV keratitis, snow blindness) is an injury to the outer layer of the cornea. Symptoms include tearing, swelling of the eyelid, pain, sensitivity to light, and blurred vision. You may feel as though a foreign body is in the eye (which should be looked for by checking under each lid). The eye may be bloodshot and red. Good polarizing sunglasses can prevent UV eye injury and should be worn when the eyes are exposed to bright sunlight during any season, but especially around sand, water, or snow. If injury is suspected, see a doctor as soon as possible. Until then, place a patch over the eye.

VOMITING

Aside from being a particularly unpleasant experience, vomiting may result in dehydration and serious chemical imbalances. Mild nausea and vomiting can be controlled by a liquid diet, with the liquids sipped almost continuously. Severe vomiting is difficult to treat without access to intravenous fluids and intramuscular injections of medications.

If vomiting is to be properly treated, the underlying cause must be determined. A great variety of problems can cause vomiting, including middle ear disease, food poisoning, acute viral infections, brain tumors, heart attacks, and bowel blockage. In the early stages, vomiting caused by some mild stomach upset may be difficult to distinguish from vomiting attributable to more serious or even life-threatening disorders.

Obviously, the safest solution is to consult a physician, who can usually determine the cause and effectively treat your problem.

Basically, vomiting without other associated symptoms is usually not serious, especially if the vomiting is short-lived. Waiting it out and a clear liquid diet may suffice.

Persistent or severe vomiting is reason for concern. The vomiting itself may lead to problems of dehydration and electrolyte imbalance, which can be particularly serious in young children, the elderly, those with chronic diseases, such as diabetes, heart disease, and kidney disease, and individuals receiving oral medication. These patients should all seek medical care.

Other symptoms, such as vertigo (the sensation of spinning), abdominal pain, headache, chest pain, diarrhea, or changes in mental state, are serious warning signals and the patient must see a physician as soon as possible. Those who vomit blood or who are very weak also fall into this category. In such seriously ill patients avoid all forms of treatment on your own; don't let the patient eat or drink; get medical help.

Prevention of nausea and vomiting is preferable to treatment. See the entry on *Motion Sickness* for tips on how to deal with this cause of vomiting. Nausea will often respond to one of the antihistamine medications, such as Vistaril. Avoiding contaminated food and water is also helpful (see *Foods* and *Water* entries). Finally, when vomiting ceases, the fluids and electrolytes lost must be replaced. Your natural appetites are good guides to how much you need to drink.

EMPHYSEMA

All patients with chronic obstructive pulmonary disease (COPD), including emphysema and bronchitis, should be under a doctor's care. Before any significant trip is considered, the potential problems associated with travel should be discussed with the physician. In patients with mild disease, extraordinary measures may be unnecessary. Those with COPD, however, should avoid smoke or other pollutants, carry antibiotics in case of a pulmonary infection, and consider receiving flu shots before traveling.

Patients with moderate to severe COPD associated with some degree of breathlessness should consult their physicians before any trip. Prescriptions should be obtained for a supply of medication sufficient for the entire trip, as well as extra prescriptions in case medication is lost. All drugs should be carried with the patient to avoid loss as well as damage by extremes in temperature.

Specifically, the patient should question the physician with regard to the advisability of travel and the safety of air travel. If the patient plans to fly and needs supplemental oxygen, the airline should be notified of this need at least forty-eight hours before flight time and again when the patient checks in. He or she should request a seat as far from the smoking area as possible. Smokers and smoking areas should also be avoided when traveling by bus, train, or car.

The patient with COPD should avoid dehydration and contact with individuals with respiratory illnesses. If a fever, productive cough, or other signs of respiratory infection develop, a physician should be consulted as soon as possible. If no doctor is available, the patient should begin taking whatever antibiotic has been prescribed by his or her physician and should consider shortening the trip.

If more physical activity than usual is planned, especially in a climate different from that at home, conditioning should be undertaken and abilities tested before leaving home. Even patients with relatively severe lung disease can train their muscles to be more efficient and thereby increase their exercise tolerance. Such conditioning ought to begin four to six weeks before embarking and should be undertaken under the direction of a doctor.

Be reasonable about your functional abilities and know what to expect. If shortness of breath occurs with little exertion at sea level, significant difficulties can be expected at high altitudes. If travel to a very high altitude is planned, make provisions for a rapid return in case altitude sickness occurs. (see *Altitude-Related Illnesses*).

EPILEPSY

The term epilepsy is used to refer to seizure disorders of various types. Thousands of individuals with epilepsy are able to travel without restrictions. The most important factor in determining the ability of an epileptic patient to travel is how well seizures are controlled. Patients receiving anticonvulsant medications who have experienced no seizures for one year or more are unlikely to have any difficulty. Patients with poorly controlled epilepsy, can achieve adequate control of seizures if a good physician is consulted and his or her advice is followed.

Before leaving on a major trip, patients with epilepsy should visit a doctor, have anticonvulsant blood levels checked, and obtain enough medication for the trip, as well as extra prescriptions in case some medication is lost. A letter explaining that the patient has epilepsy, as well as a necklace, bracelet, or wallet card identifying the patient as an epileptic, should be carried.

Certain precautions are necessary even for patients with well-controlled seizures. Medication must never be missed. Patients ought to have names of contactable doctors available at each destination. Because certain tranquilizers and other drugs can increase the chances of a seizure, patients should inform their doctors of any anti-seizure medication they may be taking. Overindulgence in alcohol or caffeine, exhaustion, loss of sleep, and missed meals should be avoided as well as any activities, such as scuba diving, in which a seizure would be life-threatening. Patients with poorly controlled seizures should not voluntarily travel, drive, or fly.

If seizures occur while traveling, medical care should be sought as soon as possible. When possible, epileptic patients should travel with a companion who knows the patient's condition and can deal with a seizure if one occurs.

FIRE

Five thousand hotel and motel fires occur each year. A certain percentage of these fires result in the death of one or more hotel guests. Although burns are responsible for some of these deaths, others are caused by inhalation of smoke or toxic gases and many are simply the result of panic. A number of steps can be taken to increase your chances of survival in the unlikely event of a hotel or motel fire.

Prevention of a hotel fire is not totally within your control. However, there are a few precautions that you can take to reduce the likelihood of a fire starting in your room. Most important of all, don't smoke in bed. When you do smoke, carefully dispose of matches and cigarettes, cigar butts, or pipe ashes. Don't abuse alcohol or sedatives to the extent that your judgment or your ability to respond to an emergency is affected.

Knowing what you would do in the event of a fire is the best method of protecting yourself. When you check into a hotel room, assume that you may have to escape and plan your route of escape.

If possible, stay in a room located no higher than the third floor. The next best location is the floor below the roof, provided that access to the roof exists.

Familiarize yourself with your room. Know the location of the windows and whether or not they open. Know where the exits are located. Check the stairway exits on your floor to make sure they are unlocked and count the number of doors to these exits. Become familiar with any objects, such as ice machines, that might obstruct your path in a dark, smoke-filled hallway. Check and locate any type of fire extinguishers near your room. Note whether or not your bathroom has a vent or window. Keep your key on the table next to your bed.

If you detect a fire, call the front desk to report it and to request information concerning its extent. Don't assume that the hotel employees will report the fire to the fire department. Obtain an outside telephone line and report the fire yourself.

At the first sign of smoke or fire, take your key and crawl on your hands and knees to the door. Touch the door with the palm of your hand; if it is hot, don't open it. If the door is not hot, open it slightly and look into the hallway. If you can, make your escape to the nearest safe exit, taking your key and closing your room door behind you. If the hall contains smoke, crawl to the exit; if no smoke is present, run. *Do not use the elevators*.

Drape a wet towel or sheet across your nose and mouth to protect your face and airways from the heat and smoke. Stay against the wall to orient yourself and to avoid being trampled by others who may be running in panic. Hold the handrail if you use the stairs. If you encounter smoke in a stairway as you descend from a higher floor, do not proceed through it. Turn around and walk back up to the roof. If the roof is not accessible, try to enter a floor that the fire has not yet reached and seek another escape route.

Never open a door that feels hot. And never panic. If all exits are blocked, take a few minutes to collect your thoughts and formulate a plan. Phone the desk to let them know that you are in your room. Hang a sheet out of your window and flash the lights to attract attention. Turn on the bathroom vent and stuff door cracks with wet cloths. Place the mattress against the door and block it with heavy furniture. Keep the door wet. Open windows to vent the smoke, unless the fire is threatening from outside the building. Remove all flammable materials from the windows. Fill the bathtub with water. Wet a towel and tie it around your mouth and nose. Swing a wet towel around the room and throw water on any fire or hot walls.

Jumping from the window or roof may also be considered as a means of escape. If your room is below the third floor, jumping feet first, taking care to avoid broken glass, window sills and ledges, may be the best alternative. If you are above the third floor, the likelihood of surviving a jump is small. Your chances are better if you take what measures you can and wait to be rescued. Above all, remain calm and use common sense. Remember that the most smokeless air is nearest to the floor.

FISH POISONING (CIGUATERA)

Fish poisoning may be caused by eating certain fish found around tropical reefs. The toxin responsible for this illness is found in the flesh, fat, and viscera of large predators, such as barracuda, grouper, and snapper. The fish probably accumulate the toxin from their diet.

Symptoms may occur within a few hours of eating the fish and include nausea, vomiting, diarrhea, numbness, weakness, abdominal pain, itching, and shock. An afflicted patient may have only a few of these symptoms. Severe poisoning can be fatal, and there is no effective first aid. Anyone suspected of having ciguatera fish poisoning should seek professional medical care as soon as possible.

FITNESS

A vacation is an excellent time to begin getting into shape; it's also an opportunity to expand your regular fitness program.

However, be sure not to overdo it; remember, it takes only twenty minutes of steady aerobic activity, three times each week to get into shape and stay that way.

If you plan to be more physically active than usual while traveling, it is advisable to get into shape before you leave home. Begin two or three weeks before your trip and continue your exercise schedule while traveling.

Choose any activity that you enjoy and that will exercise most muscle groups. Jogging, push-ups, and sit-ups can be done almost anywhere. A brisk walk or jog around each place you visit during travel will help to familiarize you with each new location while you are getting your workout.

Find out if there are appropriate and safe places to jog and exercise. Many hotels now have exercise facilities for the use of guests.

If you are unable to find appropriate places, use the Canadian Armed Forces Fitness Program, an aerobic dance routine, or your imagination.

FOODS

Infected food and drink are the most common source of infections in travelers. Pay strict attention to all you eat and drink while traveling if you expect to enjoy good health and comfort.

In many places vegetables are contaminated by being grown in soil in which infected human or animal feces has been used as fertilizer. Vegetables and fruit are often washed in water containing dangerous bacteria. Nonpasteurized milk, as well as cheese or other dairy products made from raw milk, may carry a host of infections. Meat may be infected with parasites or contaminated with bacteria caused by lack of refrigeration. As a rule of thumb, remember that these foods are usually safe in English-speaking countries but suspect in most other places unless you have information to the contrary. The best guides to follow are the publications by IAMAT that outline the safety of meats, vegetables, fruit, milk, and milk and water products in various cities (see *IAMAT*).

In order to make contaminated food safe, it must be adequately cooked. Raw fruits have surface contamination but removing the peel will make the fruit safe; peel it yourself after you have washed your hands in safe water. Breads are usually safe, but toasting adds some factor of safety.

Sealed beverages are usually safe if they are name brands, especially if they are international products. Some local beverages may be made with contaminated water and are unsafe. Alcoholic beverages are usually safe.

(See entries *Milk*, *Water*, and *IAMAT*.)

FOREIGN TRAVELERS TO THE UNITED STATES

Travelers to the United States have access to some of the best medical care in the world. Unfortunately, it is also the most expensive care in the world. Emergency outpatient care by a private physician may not constitute an extreme financial burden to travelers to the U.S., but hospitalization, with or without surgery, can be a financial catastrophe because most non-U.S. health policies do not cover care in this country. Fortunately, good and relatively inexpensive health insurance can be purchased for the duration of your trip. Such insurance is recommended for all travelers to the United States.

Travelers to the U.S., as well as to any other country, should be sure to have health and accident insurance coverage. *Business Traveler* magazine recommends Extrasure and also mentions that Tugu, Blue Cross, Taikoo and Malayan are useful policies. Most such policies can be purchased through insurance agents. Extrasure uses Medex International Corporation for handling claims. In addition to coverage, Medex offers a number of other extras, including approved lists of doctors and hospitals, and a consulting service that will assist travelers in deciding whether they should seek medical care where they are or elsewhere. This latter service may be most valuable in developing countries, or areas notorious for poor and even dangerous medical care.

In most industrialized countries, including the United States, accidents are one of the leading causes of injury and death. Common sense, avoidance of intoxication by alcohol or drugs, and the use of seat belts can go a very long way toward insuring a safe, trauma-free trip.

FUNGAL INFECTIONS

Desert fever or valley fever (coccidioidomycosis) is an acute flulike illness caused by a fungus found in the southwestern part of the United States. Desert fever has been known to affect residents of and visitors to Arizona, New Mexico, Texas, the San Joaquin Valley in California, and parts of Nevada and Utah. The disease is also found in Mexico, Guatemala, Nicaragua, Venezuela, Colombia, Paraguay and Argentina. The infection is believed to be caused by inhalation of the fungus from the soil and cannot be communicated by personal contact.

Symptoms of desert fever develop within approximately ten to fourteen days after exposure to the fungus. These symptoms include fever, chest pain, dry cough, muscular aches, fatigue, and lethargy and may persist for up to six months. Other than avoiding areas where the fungus is found, especially during dust storms, no preventive measures exist. The disease is self-limited in 95% of all cases. Physicians in areas in which desert fever is endemic are usually aware of this illness, but physicians in regions where the disease is uncommon may not recognize the symptoms unless they are informed of your recent travels.

Histoplasmosis is a similar illness caused by a different type of fungus that is found in the east central part of the United States, especially in the Mississippi and Missouri river valleys.

If a flulike respiratory illness should develop while traveling in an area in which fungal infections are known to occur, contact a physician to determine if you have influenza or one of these fungal diseases.

GLASSES AND CONTACT LENSES

Travelers who require vision correction should be sure to pack at least one extra pair of glasses or contact lenses. Don't forget to bring your prescription sunglasses whenever you travel. If you plan to be more physically active than usual, obtain glasses with unbreakable lenses and purchase a head cord to hold your glasses on. Also carry the refraction prescription for your lenses.

GUIDE DOGS

Blindness need not bar travel anymore than it prevents other daily functions. While traveling on commercial carriers, the blind should identify themselves to attendants so that they can be advised of unannounced seat-belt and smoking conditions. Those with guide dogs should seek a window seat, when possible, for the convenience of the other passengers.

Guide dogs are permitted in the cabin of airplanes on most, but not all, flights. The policy of the airlines should be determined before reservations are made. Certain countries will not permit guide dogs to enter, and flights to these countries will not allow guide dogs aboard. These countries include Australia,

Hong Kong, Ireland, New Zealand, and the United Kingdom. The state of Hawaii also does not allow guide dogs aboard flights. Canada allows guide dogs to enter the country without any medical certification, but many other countries have strict regulations concerning dogs. Some countries, including Sweden, Norway, and Denmark, require certification of rabies vaccine. Others require a veterinarian's certificate stating that the dog is free of rabies, rabies exposure, and other infections. Norway even requires an examination by a veterinarian at the airport before the dog is allowed to enter. It is best to call or write the embassies of any countries to be visited and to check with the commercial carrier before embarking on a trip abroad with a dog. Otherwise, you may be refused entrance to a country or find your dog quarantined for weeks or even months.

HEARING AID

Travelers with hearing aids should bring spare batteries and if possible, an extra hearing aid.

HEART DISEASE

The stress of traveling may aggravate certain heart diseases. If you have heart disease or the risk factors associated with heart disease (smoking, high blood pressure, diabetes, high cholesterol level, obesity, a family history of heart disease, type A personality, sedentary life-style) see your physician and have an ECG done before you travel. Carry a copy of your ECG with you for comparison.

Chest pain is a common symptom of heart disease and always demands medical attention. At times the pain of coronary artery disease may also be felt in the neck, jaw, arms, hands, upper abdomen, or upper back, in addition to, or instead of, the chest. Other symptoms suggestive of heart disease are shortness of breath (especially with exertion or when lying flat), palpitations, or short episodes of loss of consciousness. Should any of these symptoms occur while traveling, remain calm and go to the nearest emergency facility. Bring your ECG from home with you for the doctor to examine and compare.

If you have heart disease and plan to exert yourself during a trip, attempt a similar level of exertion at home before you leave. It is better to determine your limitations at home rather than en route to or in a foreign area. Discuss your planned activity with your doctor before your trip.

HEAT-RELATED PROBLEMS

A body temperature of approximately 98.6° F is needed for proper functioning. Heat is produced primarily by muscle activity and liver function. The heat is dissipated by the blood as it passes through the skin; evaporation of sweat also results in a cooling effect. In order to cool the body and prevent fever at very warm temperatures, the heart must work harder in order to pump more blood to the skin's surface. For effective perspiration and adequate cooling, there must be sufficient fluid in the body. The body, performing these cooling functions, becomes more efficient with continuous exposure to warm environments; it adjusts to the heat over a period of time.

Heat-related problems are a result of excess heat production or insufficient cooling, or both. Vigorous exercise may produce excess heat or hot humid weather may prevent efficient evaporation of sweat. The final result is an increased body temperature with accompanying malfunction. Certain medications can interfere with cooling and aggravate these conditions. Heat exhaustion is one relatively common heat-related disorder. The blood pressure decreases, although the temperature may be normal or only slightly elevated. The victim may feel weak, thirsty, exhausted, and light-headed. Eventually, if cooling does not occur, the afflicted individual becomes delirious and may lose consciousness. Sweating occurs in case of heat exhaustion, but if fluid intake is insufficient, dehydration may occur, resulting in decreased sweating and a rise in body temperature. A more severe problem called heatstroke (sunstroke) occurs when the temperature rises. Sweating is no longer present, and mental changes occur. If left untreated, the patient may become comatose, sustain brain injury, and even die.

Less severe effects of heat include swollen ankles and feet, as well as muscle cramps. Heat cramps appear as a cramping pain in the large muscles, such as the calves, thighs, or abdominal muscles.

Prevention of the heat-related disorders is preferable to treatment. If long-term exposure to heat is anticipated, it may take four to six weeks for the body to become completely acclimated. In the meantime, fluid and salt intake should be increased and vigorous exercise avoided. At temperatures below 67° F there is little danger of heat-related problems, but the risk increases as the temperature rises above 67° F. Increased humidity is also a risk factor. When temperature and humidity are both over 78° F, the risks are considerable, especially in individuals who are exercising.

When the temperature and humidity are high, wear loose cotton clothing and be sure to cover arms, legs, and head to avoid overexposure to the sun. Pay attention to early symptoms, such as fatigue, chills, dizziness, headache, or nausea. At the first sign of problems, stop exercising, go to a cool place, and take fluids. If symptoms persist or increase, cool off with cold water, wet towels, fans, or even ice and consult a doctor.

Individuals with heart disease and the very young and very old are more vulnerable to heat-related problems. Those with a past history of heatstroke may also be more vulnerable. Those who take the following medications and/or drugs are prone to heatstroke: aspirin, cocaine, antihistamines, PCP, alcohol, tranquilizers, antidepressants, LSD, and amphetamines. Certain extensive skin diseases that interfere with sweating may also contribute to heat-related problems.

In summary, heat-related problems can be avoided by limiting physical exercise in hot, humid weather and by drinking plenty of fluids. At the first sign of illness, stop exercising, cool yourself, and drink fluids. If severe illness occurs, seek medical care.

HEAT DISORDERS

	Symptoms	Treatment
Heat Cramps	Gastrocnemius spasms 60%	Rest
	Thigh spasms 30%	Ice packs on muscles
	Other muscle spasms 10%	Application of pressure to muscle
		Water replacement

Heat Syncope	Weakness	Cessation of activity
	Tiredness	Removal from direct sunlight
	Dizziness	Application of iced towels
	Weak, rapid pulse	Water replacement
	Decreased blood pressure	
Heat Exhaustion	Extreme weakness	Cooling of body
	Exhaustion	Fluid replacement with cool or cold liquids
	Unconsciousness sometimes	Electrolyte replacement
	Profuse sweating	Hospitalization if patients is unconscious or vomiting
	Normal or slightly elevated body temperatures	
	Thirst	
	Oliguria (little urination)	
	Giddiness (often euphoria)	
	Delirium	
Heatstroke	Faintness	Rapid cooling of body with ice packs, iced towels, cold tub bath
	Dizziness	
	Staggering	Hospitalization if necessary
	Headache	
	Nausea	Sedation by physician with chlorpromazine and promethazine hydrochloride
	Confusion or unconsciousness	
	High body temperature	Rapid fluid replacement
	Strong, rapid pulse	
	Hot, dry skin	

HIKING

Hiking is an ideal, healthful form of outdoor activity, and almost anyone who is ambulatory can probably handle some level of hiking with relative comfort and safety. Most healthy individuals are capable of walking up to 10 miles over several hours without a pack. Anyone considering a hike in remote or inaccessible areas is advised to take a comparably long walk around home first to be sure that they are physically able. Those unaccustomed to walking will sometimes experience muscle aches and pains and some blisters. It is best to learn to deal with these problems before embarking on a hiking trip.

Hiking more than 10 miles or over rocky surfaces or hiking with a pack is more than just a walk in the woods. It is hard physical exercise and is not to be taken lightly by anyone who is not well and physically fit. Individuals with heart disease, lung problems, blood-vessel disease, physical disabilities, or any other serious illness should discuss any strenuous hiking plans with their physicians. If your doctor approves, start a program of physical exercise to condition yourself for the hike; progressively longer trails should be part of your program. This approach will maximize the safety and pleasure of this activity. Unfit and unwell persons certainly do hike without preparation, but this approach sometimes results in great discomfort or even physical injury and turns what should be an enjoyable experience into an unpleasant one.

Older, comfortable, well-fitting shoes are your most important item. Footwear need not be expensive but should be appropriate for the conditions you expect to encounter. Running shoes are great for firm terrain in relatively warm weather but are inappropriate for long hikes in snow. Do not buy new footwear and then go on a long hike; cramps and blisters are sure to develop. Break in footwear gradually and wear socks that fit well. On long hikes, have at least one extra pair of walking shoes and dry socks. Prevention is far superior to treatment of blisters, sore feet, bunions, or athlete's foot. If you have difficulties with your feet, consult a podiatrist for treatment and advice before you begin hiking.

Clothing should be appropriate for the conditions. The concept of layering is useful because you can peel off clothing as you warm up and add it when you cool down. Regard your pack, if you carry one, as part of your clothing. Use your pack while you condition for any long hikes so that any problems, such as shoulder discomfort or skin irritation from straps, can be dealt with before your trip.

Travel as lightly as possible, but don't forget essential medication for any existing illness. If the hike promises to be a long one, take along a medical kit (described on p. 5). Other useful items include sunscreen, insect repellent, gloves, rain gear, and extra glasses.

HOMOSEXUALS

Homosexuals have some special problems concerning sexually-transmitted diseases and other illnesses. In addition to the usual sexually-transmitted diseases experienced by heterosexuals, they also have a high incidence of hepatitis B (serum hepatitis), rectal gonorrhea, pharyngeal gonorrhea and unusual diseases such as AIDS, Kaposi's sarcoma, toxoplasmosis and rectal herpes. Therefore, homosexuals who develop an illness while traveling should be sure to inform their doctors about their homosexual contacts as well as the countries in which these contacts occurred. (See *Sexually-Transmitted Diseases*.)

HYPNOSIS

Hypnosis can be a very useful aid to the traveler. Almost anyone who can be hypnotized can be taught to use self-hypnosis.

During long waits or anxiety-producing situations such as rough flights, self-relaxation can turn unpleasant phases of travel into restful or exciting experiences. The concentration learned in hypnosis can help you absorb and appreciate what you might otherwise miss. The relaxation techniques are helpful in achieving sleep and relaxation in the face of unfamiliar surroundings and unusual schedules.

Additionally, hypnosis may help you cope with personal fears that can interfere with travel. Hypnosis can help conquer fear of flying, fear of heights, and fear of water.

INFANTS

Traveling with infants need not be much more complicated than caring for them at home. However, traveling with a sick infant can be a great burden and is not encouraged. Sometimes it may be necessary to take a sick infant on a trip, but, with proper planning and knowledge, difficulties can be avoided.

First, check your intended destinations (see p. 105) for the rules and recommendations concerning vaccinations which may differ for infants and adults. Also check the appropriate entries on modes of travel (*Air Travel, Automobiles, Seas and Ships*). Although many states have laws requiring special restraints for infants traveling by auto, infants should be properly restrained or belted whenever they travel in cars, whether or not the law requires it. Have infants drink when taking off and landing in an airplane. Because infants are especially vulnerable to many infectious and diarrheal diseases, strictly follow the recommendations concerning safe food and water.

Sick infants should be examined by a physician before traveling. Discuss your trip with the physician and ask his or her advice concerning special preparations and recommendations.

Airlines and other commercial carriers will usually go out of their way to assist you with infants. Notify the carrier of your needs and ask what assistance is offered, such as early boarding, special foods, and special seating. Check in early if you require assistance.

Join IAMAT, the International Association of Medical Assistance to Travellers, if you plant to travel to developing countries (see *IAMAT*). Their current list of worldwide English-speaking physicians could be a life saver for your infant while traveling.

INFECTIOUS DISEASES IN THE U.S.

Alabama	RMSF (Rocky Mountain Spotted Fever)
Alaska	
Arizona	rattlesnake, scorpion, coral snake, Gila monster, black widow, plague
Arkansas	Lyme
California	Lyme, plague, RMSF, Colorado tick fever, murine typhus, trachoma
Colorado	RMSF, anthrax, Colorado tick fever
Connecticut	Lyme, RMSF
Delaware	RMSF, Lyme
Florida	RMSF, Lyme

Georgia	RMSF, Lyme
Hawaii	murine typhus
Idaho	RMSF, Colorado tick fever
Illinois	RMSF
Indiana	RMSF
Iowa	RMSF
Kansas	RMSF, typhus
Kentucky	RMSF
Louisiana	typhus, cholera
Maine	
Maryland	Lyme, RMSF, typhus
Massachusetts	babesiasis (Martha's Vinyard, Nantucket), Lyme, RMSF
Michigan	RMSF
Minnesota	Lyme
Mississippi	RMSF
Missouri	RMSF
Montana	scorpion, RMSF, Colorado tick fever
Nebraska	RMSF
Nevada	plague
New Hampshire	
New Jersey	Lyme, RMSF
New Mexico	plague, scorpion, Colorado tick fever
New York	Lyme (Westchester County, Shelter Island, Long Island), babesiosis (Long Island, Fire Island)
North Carolina	RMSF
North Dakota	
Ohio	RMSF, Colorado tick fever, typhus
Oklahoma	RMSF
Oregon	scorpion, Lyme, RMSF, Colorado tick fever, plague
Pennsylvania	RMSF, typhus, Lyme
Rhode Island	RMSF, typhus, Lyme
South Carolina	RMSF, typhus
South Dakota	RMSF, Colorado tick fever
Tennessee	RMSF, typhus
Texas	RMSF, scorpion, murine typhus, Lyme, plague (west)
Utah	RMSF, Colorado tick fever
Vermont	
Virginia	RMSF, typhus
Washington	scorpion, typhus, Colorado tick fever, plague
West Virginia	Lyme, RMSF
Wisconsin	Lyme
Wyoming	RMSF, Colorado tick fever, plague

(IAMAT) INTERNATIONAL ASSOCIATION FOR MEDICAL ASSISTANCE TO TRAVELLERS

The IAMAT, established in 1960, offers very valuable services to travelers, free of charge. One of the most valuable services is the free, annually-updated directory of physicians that lists competent, English-speaking physicians in over 450 cities throughout the world. These physicians are available to IAMAT members twenty-four hours a day, seven days a week, at a fixed fee (currently between $20 and $35). If you become ill while traveling, this list of doctors, reprinted at the end of this book, could be the most valuable item in your suitcase.

Another valuable service is their publication of twenty-four world climate charts covering over 1400 locations throughout the world. These charts are well worth your $15 donation. Each chart lists climate information for each month at any given location, including average temperatures, humidity, and number of rainy days, together with suggestions on what type of clothing to bring and wear. Altitude for each site is provided in both meters and feet. Even more important is the information in these charts concerning the safety of water, dairy products, and uncooked food.

Other helpful publications provided by IAMAT include:

Traveller Clinical Record
World Immunization Chart
World Malaria Risk Chart
World Schistosomiasis Risk Chart
How to Adjust to Heat
How to Adapt to Altitude
How to Protect Yourself Against Malaria

To join IAMAT, write:
IAMAT
736 Center Street
Lewiston, NY 14092

There is no charge for joining IAMAT, but contributions are accepted and appreciated.

JET LAG

Jet lag is the term used to describe the discomfort that is frequently associated with rapid travel through multiple time zones.

The symptoms of jet lag may include nervousness, depression, fatigue, irritability, insomnia, drowsiness, and a host of other complaints difficult to describe and unpleasant to endure. Some of the symptoms included in jet lag may be attributed to the physical and emotional stresses of travel as well as to the disruption of meals and sleep. Overindulgence in alcohol, food, or caffeine, as well as the effects of sleeping pills, sedatives, or other drugs may add to the traveler's discomfort. The symptoms of jet lag may unfavorably influence a vacation or business trip, and any measures that will help to alleviate the symptoms associated with this phenomenon are warranted.

The cause of jet lag is thought to be a disruption in the body's circadian rhythm, an internal chemical, clocklike mechanism. The hormone blood levels and other body chemicals vary with the time of day. The levels of these agents are appropriately adjusted for sleeping, meals, rest, and activity. When a change occurs in the timing of these various activities, the levels of these chemicals must change accordingly. Unfortunately, these adjustments may take days to occur. The time required for the body to make these chemical adjustments is related to the degree of disruption of the usual behavior pattern.

The number of days required for the body to adjust naturally to a time change depends on the direction of travel and the number of time zones through which the traveler has passed. Travel north or south in the same time zone is not associated with jet lag. Travel from east to west across the time zones is likely to be associated with a lesser degree of jet lag than travel from west to east. The number of days needed to fully adjust also varies from person to person. In general, however, traveling east usually requires one day for each time zone passed. Traveling west may require one or two days less than the number of time zones.

Other than letting nature take its course, there are at least three methods of minimizing symptoms of jet lag. First, a few days before departing on your trip, you can begin to change the time of your meals and your sleep cycle to correspond with those you will face at your destination. For example, before heading east, go to bed progressively later for a few days preceding the trip, arise later, and have your meals closer to the times that you will have them at your destination. An alternative approach is to refuse to deviate from your regular cycle. Keep your watch at the same time as your point of departure and continue to eat your meals and sleep at your normal time. Both of these methods, however, may be difficult for anyone who must function and interact with others in a work situation.

A relatively new approach is described in the book *Overcoming Jet Lag* by Charles F. Ehret and Lynne Waller Scanlon (Berkley, $4.95). This program, developed by the Argonne National Laboratory, and used by President Ronald Reagan, on his trip to China, recommends alternating days of heavy eating or feasting with days of light eating or fasting before departing on a trip. Breakfast and lunch consist of high-protein foods, whereas supper is very high in carbohydrates. Caffeine is avoided or, if used at all, is consumed only at specific times, for example, in the morning when traveling west and in the evening when traveling east. No alcohol is allowed during the flight. Ideally the trip should be planned so that upon arrival you will sleep until breakfast and then begin your day with a heavy breakfast. If you arrive in the daylight, however, you should stay up. Such a program has been claimed to minimize jet lag considerably and will decrease the time required to adjust to a new time zone. Travelers using this method may need only three days to adjust to a new time zone, even when they have passed through eleven or twelve time zones.

Other measures that may help to minimize jet lag include sleeping, or at least resting, during periods of darkness, and staying up during hours of daylight, avoiding alcohol as well as caffeine, and eating when you are hungry but never to the point of feeling full. Walking as much as possible, at least hourly during waking hours, during a long flight, may also be helpful.

TIPS FOR DEALING WITH JET LAG

- Don't overindulge in food or drink during travel.
- Avoid alcohol and caffeine during travel.
- Begin readjusting meals and sleeping patterns before departure.
- Begin eating high-protein breakfast and lunch and high-carbohydrate supper four days before departure.
- Alternate days of fasting and feasting.

- During flight and upon arrival, sleep or rest during periods of darkness and stay up and active during daylight hours.
- Get adequate rest before the trip.
- Exercise regularly before and during the trip.
- Travel from east to west whenever possible.
- Recognize jet lag and realize it is temporary.

LEPROSY

Leprosy is caused by an organism closely related to the tuberculosis bacillus. Although leprosy is found all over the world, it poses no threat to travelers. It is transmitted only to very close contacts of active cases, and even then only 5% of close family members develop leprosy, usually only after many years. Visits to leprosariums can be made safely; the only precaution required is to wash your hands after touching a patient with leprosy.

LYME DISEASE

Lyme disease is an illness transmitted by ticks during their spring, summer, and fall periods of activity. It was originally described in Lyme, Connecticut, but is now seen in Australia, Europe (Switzerland, Germany, France), Canada (Ontario, British Columbia) and in at least fourteen states (Arkansas, California, Connecticut, Delaware, Georgia, Massachusetts, Minnesota, New Jersey, New York, Oregon, Pennsylvania, Rhode Island, Wisconsin and Texas).

A small red lump develops two to fourteen days after a tick bite and subsequently spreads. The rash may involve more than one area and is frequently warm and tender and may itch. Many of the patients also have painful swollen joints, usually knees or the large joints. In a few patients, joint pain alone or rash alone is the only manifestation of the disease. Other symptoms include fever, fatigue, headache, stiff neck, and muscle aches. Less commonly, patients develop numbness or weakness after the rash clears. Symptoms may persist for months in some patients. Early treatment with penicillin or tetracycline may decrease the joint pains.

Lyme disease may be prevented by avoiding tick-infested areas. Regular tick inspection and removal of ticks while traveling in infected areas will offer some protection. Protective clothing and insect repellents also offer protection, although tick inspections are still required. (See *Ticks* under *Bites and Stings*.)

MALARIA

Definition: Parasitic disease contracted from mosquitoes (anopheles) and associated with periodic high fevers, chills, sweats and headaches.

Explanation: There are a number of different species of malaria (Plasmodium) all of which attack the red blood cells. Most forms (except Plasmodium falciparum) also involve the liver. Delayed attacks may occur in some form (Vivax, Ovale) many months after leaving an infected area.

Avoidance: Stay away from malaria areas (almost all are tropical) to prevent exposure to mosquitoes infected with malaria.

Sleeping under mosquito netting at night and staying in well screened areas during mosquito feeding times (usually evening, but ask the local residents) can decrease the chances of infection. Wear protective clothing in malaria areas. Liberally use insect repellents on clothes and body. The most effective repellents contain deet (N-N-diethyl-meta-toluomide).

Preventive treatment is recommended by the U.S. Public Health Service for all travelers to areas where malaria exists. Conditions and risks change but malaria is found in parts of Mexico, Haiti, Central America, South America, Africa, the Middle East, Turkey, India, China, Indonesia, and Oceania.

Medications: *Chloroquine phosphate.* Standard dosage: If weight is above 50 kg (110 pounds), 500 mg once a week; if weight is less than 50 kg, 5 mg (base) per kilogram. Taken one week before, during, and for six weeks after travel to areas with malaria, taken by all those exposed, all ages.

WORLD DISTRIBUTION OF MALARIA

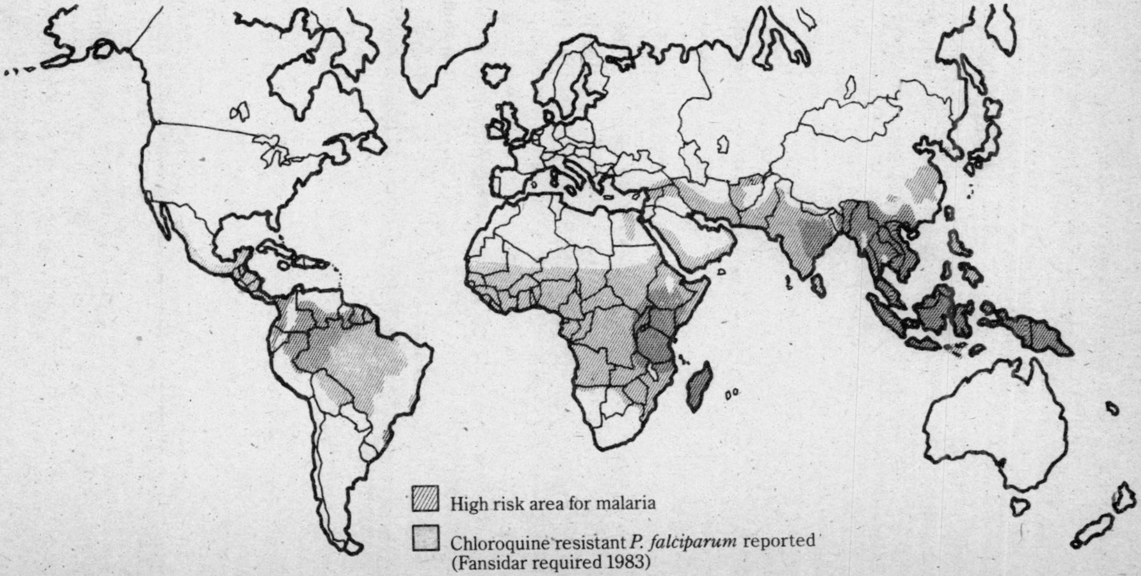

Pyrimethamine/sulfadoxine Fansidar. Standard dosage: One tablet once a week in addition to chloroquine phosphate, if in areas with *P. falciparum* resistant to chloroquine phosphate (e.g., East Africa, parts of South America, Panama, Indonesia, the Philippines, and New Guinea).

Primaquine. Useful in some specific situations; check with physician; not for pregnant women.

(Some strains of malaria are resistant both to chloroquine phosphate and pyrimethamine/sulfadoxine.)

MEASLES

Measles occurs worldwide but it is becoming much less common in the United States. Most adult U.S. travelers born before 1957 are probably immune to this disease. Those born after 1957 who are not immune (individuals are considered immune if measles was diagnosed by a physician—a blood test provides evidence of previous measles—or a live virus measles vaccine was given after age one) should receive a measles vaccine before traveling. The disease is highly contagious and can cause serious complications and death, especially in infants and adults. Persons who received measles vaccine (which was used between 1963 and 1967) should be revaccinated before traveling outside of the United States. Check with your physician.

MEDIC ALERT FOUNDATION INTERNATIONAL

This nonprofit organization provides medical identification in the form of metal disks attached to a bracelet or necklace. The patient's medical problem is engraved on the disk along with an emergency telephone number which can be called collect from nearly any place in the world. Operators provide important health information concerning the patient as identified by the membership number on the metal disk.

Medic Alert is especially recommended for travelers with

specific severe allergies, diabetes, pacemakers, Addison's disease, epilepsy, myasthenia gravis, and for those taking certain medications, such as anticoagulants or hydrocortisone. Such information could be life saving for a traveler who is found unconscious or incapacitated. Emergency personnel frequently search for a Medic Alert disk when confronted with such a patient.

In order to join, send $15.00 to

Medic Alert Foundation International
Department AZ
P. O. Box 1009
Turlock, CA 95381.

Their telephone number is 800-344-3226. Operators are on duty twenty-four hours each day; French and Spanish interpreters are available.

Any traveler with a serious disease should seriously consider wearing a Medic Alert disk. This is especially so for those who travel alone.

MILK AND MILK PRODUCTS

Milk and products made from milk carry infectious organisms if the milk has not been pasteurized. Do not ingest such products in areas where there is any question about pasteurization. Raw milk can never be presumed to be safe. Although many travelers avoid milk, they tend to be less careful about cheese. Cheeses or milk can transmit the following diseases:

Brucellosis (nonspecific febrile illness)

Streptococcus (group C) infection

Staphylococcus infection (enteritis with vomiting and diarrhea

Salmonella (diarrheal disease)

Tuberculosis of bowel and lymph nodes

Camylobacter infection (diarrheal disease)

E. coli infection (diarrheal disease).

Generally, in developing countries where water is unsafe, so is the milk. World climate charts from IAMAT (see entry on *IAMAT*) indicate where milk is pasteurized. All English-speaking and most developed countries require pasteurization.

MOTION SICKNESS

Motion sickness may occur while traveling in any type of vehicle. Individuals vary in their susceptibility, but most persons will experience motion sickness sometime during travel. Individual susceptibility also varies with the mode of transportation, for example, a person who becomes seasick may be able to travel by plane with no discomfort.

The symptoms of motion sickness are nausea, light-headedness, vomiting, an unsteady gait, and general malaise. Several medications exist that may be useful in preventing or decreasing the symptoms of motion sickness if taken *before travel*. Some of these medications are listed below. All may cause drowsiness. Your doctor should be consulted before using any of these drugs.

Dimenhydrinate (Dramamine) is an antihistamine that may be obtained without a prescription. The first tablet should be taken 30 to 60 minutes before beginning a trip. Thereafter, one tablet may be taken every four hours as needed.

Meclizine (Antivert, Bonine) is another antihistamine that should also be taken 30 to 60 minutes before travel. Only one tablet per day is required.

Promethazine (Phenergan) is a phenothiazine derivative with antihistamine properties.

Scopolamine (Transderm-Scop) is a disk applied behind the ear that continuously releases medication. This drug may be useful during sea voyages or when nausea and vomiting prevent the use of oral medications. Some medical conditions, such as glaucoma and prostatic enlargement, are worsened by this drug.

The best approach to the treatment of motion sickness is to stop traveling. When this solution is impractical, the medications used for preventing motion sickness may be used. Reclining quietly, preferably in a cool place, and sipping chilled liquids may also be helpful.

Once travel stops, the symptoms of motion sickness will gradually disappear with time. Once you have experienced motion sickness conditions, however, you are likely to develop them again under similar conditions and preventive measures are advisable before embarking on subsequent trips.

PACEMAKER

Individuals with properly functioning pacemakers can usually travel without concern. Consult your doctor before leaving and have your pacemaker checked. If your pacemaker is being monitored by telephone, you will usually be able to do so while traveling.

Most authorities recommend that persons with pacemakers avoid scuba diving because of the danger of becoming unconscious while diving. Discuss with your physician any activities in which you wish to engage. Learn to recognize problems with your pacemaker and, if possible, travel with a responsible companion who can obtain medical help if you become disabled. Fainting episodes, weakness, or palpitations may indicate pacemaker problems.

PARASITIC DISEASES

Parasitic diseases may be transmitted by various means, such as fecal contamination of food or drink, insect bites, direct penetration of intact skin, or contamination of wounds with crushed insect debris. A knowledge of where parasites may be found and how parasitic diseases are transmitted is helpful in protecting yourself from these communicable diseases.

Some parasitic diseases are not limited to a specific area of the world. A partial list of parasites found in more than one region includes ascaris (roundworm), cysticeris, coccidia, *Echinococcus*, *Enterobius* (pinworm), *Giardia*, Balantidium, Fascioloides, hookworms, cutaneous larva migrans, *Strongyloidea*, tapeworms, *Trichinella*, Trichuris, (whipworm), Paragonimus, toxoplasma, and Pneumocystis.

Other parasites seem to be confined to specific geographic locations. For example, in the Pacific are found Angiostrongyos (the southeast), Capillaria (Philippines), or *Schistosoma japonicum* (Philippines). In the Soviet Union, the fish tapeworm, Trichostrongylus, Opisthorchias (Siberia), and *Leishmania donovani*, the cause of kala-azar (also found in the Mediterranean), may be encountered.

Parasitic diseases are most prevalent in South America, Africa, and the Orient. Many are treatable. The diagnosis of these conditions may be relatively straightforward for professionals in areas where these diseases are endemic, but may be very difficult for physicians elsewhere. Always be sure to tell your physician about your travels if symptoms should appear after you return home. If you become ill in a foreign country, a local physician may be helpful in diagnosing a local disease.

Drinking contaminated water can result in infection with Dracunculus and hookworm. Contaminated vegetables may transmit angiostrongyliasis (commonly caused by lettuce) and fascioliasis (often carried by water plants, such as watercress).

In certain Oriental countries like Japan, raw fish is consumed regularly. The following parasites may be present in raw fish: Capillaria (maribe), clonorchis (fresh water fish), fish tapeworm (fresh water fish), Gnathostoma (mullet), Anisaki (salmon, herring, cod), Heterophyes, Metagonimus, and Opisthorchis. Raw shellfish may cause typhoid, cholera, hepatitis, and viral diarrhea as well as the parasitic disease of angiostrongyliasis (shrimp) and Paragonimus (crab, crayfish). Angiostrongyliasis may also be contracted by eating raw water or land slugs or snails.

When consumed raw or served undercooked, red meats may transmit trichinosis, tapeworm, or toxoplasmosis.

When traveling, be sure to ask what you are eating and whether or not it has been cooked. Sampling new and interesting foods can be fun, but it can also make you sick. Use common sense, and follow the rules outlined in the entry *Diarrhea*.

PLAGUE

Plague is an infection carried by rodents that can be transmitted to humans through flea bites or by direct contact with infected animals. The devastating plague epidemics of history are no longer a problem, but isolated cases do occur in humans, even in the United States. Antibiotic treatment is available, but the mortality is still nearly 20%. Approximately seven cases occur each year in the U.S., all in the West, where many rodents, such as squirrels and prairie dogs, carry the plague bacillus.

Symptoms of plague usually include fever and pain in the groin or under the arms. The lymph glands in these areas are usually swollen, and pneumonia may develop. Anyone in an infected area who experiences these symptoms should consult a doctor. If no physician is available and the likelihood of infection is great, taking an antibiotic may be advisable. Tetracycline is one effective oral antibiotic for treating plague.

Most human cases of plague in the U.S. occur in parts of Arizona, Colorado, Utah, New Mexico, California, Oregon, and Nevada. If you become ill after visiting any of these areas, be sure to inform your doctor of the trip.

PREGNANCY

Pregnancy need not necessarily interfere with traveling. Thousands of pregnant women travel daily without difficulty, but if you are pregnant and planning to travel, check with your obstetrician first to ask about special precautions. Certain vaccines are not considered safe during pregnancy (see *Vaccines*).

TIPS FOR PREGNANT TRAVELERS

- Discuss the dates, places, modes of travel, vaccines and medications with your obstetrician.
- When traveling by commercial carriers, such as airlines, inform the airline personnel of your pregnant status. Avoid airplane travel after your eighth month of pregnancy.
- Certain prophylactic medications should be avoided. Do not take prophylactic antibiotics to prevent diarrhea. Do not take Fansidar.
- Malaria areas with chloroquine-resistant malaria should be avoided; if unavoidable, take only chloroquine prophylaxis.
- Have a list of physicians and/or medical facilities where you may go if medical or obstetrical problems arise.
- Do not wear your seat belt over your abdomen while driving. The lap belt should cross your pelvis or thighs.
- Avoid unnecessary travel late in pregnancy or if you are having complications or difficulties with your pregnancy.
- Avoid all medications and take only those prescribed or approved by your own obstetrician.

RABIES

Rabies is a uniformly fatal disease caused by a virus and usually transmitted by the bite of a rabid animal. Cave explorers who have inhaled the virus in caves inhabited by rabid bats have also contracted rabies. Human infections are rare in the United States, but animal rabies is not uncommon, especially in wild animals. In the U.S., any bites from bats, skunks, foxes, or raccoons should be presumed to constitute exposure to rabies unless proven otherwise by laboratory examination of the tissues from the animal.

Outside of the U.S., dog bites are commonly the cause of human rabies, especially in Mexico, South America, Africa, and Asia. A history of vaccination of domestic animals and even negative laboratory tests from suspect animals are not always reliable indicators of safety in other countries.

Recently in the U.S., cats have been found to have a higher incidence of rabies than dogs, most likely because of encounters with rabid wild animals. Rabies is almost never transmitted by rodent bites.

For most travelers, rabies is not a significant risk. However, the occasional American who develops rabies usually acquires it outside of the States. Anyone over one year of age who will be spending significant time in the bush, woods, or countryside of developing countries should consider pre-exposure rabies immunization with human diploid cell rabies vaccine (HDCV). In the high-risk areas, even those who have received pre-exposure inoculations should be given the vaccine and rabies immunoglobulin (Hyperabl) after bites by a potentially rabid animal. The new vaccine is much safer and more effective than the older vaccines and calls for only three to five relatively painless inoculations in contrast to the older painful abdominal injections.

Pre-exposure inoculations with HDCV are advised for workers assigned to or travelers planning a prolonged (longer than two weeks) visit to:

Bangladesh
Chad
Ethiopia
Guinea-Bissau
Indonesia
Morocco
Mozambique
Nepal
Nigeria
Pakistan
Philippines
Sierra Leone
Sri Lanka
Sudan
Swaziland
Tanzania
Thailand
Uganda
Upper Volta
Vietnam
Yemen

Anyone bitten by a domestic or wild animal should contact a local physician for treatment. (See *Bites*)

ROCKY MOUNTAIN SPOTTED FEVER

(See *Bites and Stings)*

SALMONELLA AND SHIGELLA

Salmonella and shigella are bacteria that may infect the bowel. Symptoms of such infections include diarrhea and occasionally fever with systemic symptoms. Infection occurs by ingestion of contaminated food or drink (frequently water). Physicians usually treat shigella infection but may elect not to treat salmonella carriers. Diagnosis is made by special cultures of stool specimens. Diarrhea that begins during or after a trip may be caused by one of these bacteria; be sure to tell your physician about your trip.

Prevention is the most effective measure (See *Diarrhea*). If one person in a group is found to be infected, other group members should have a stool check. Carriers should not handle food or drink that will be consumed by others.

SCHISTOSOMIASIS

Schistosomiasis is a parasitic disease caused by a number of different blood flukes that live in the blood vessels of animals and humans. These diseases are found in subtropical and tropical areas. Various organs can be affected, and symptoms will depend on which organ systems are infested. Infection occurs through intact skin after exposure to infected water. Human excretion from infected patients contaminates the water, but certain snails must inhabit the water in order to complete the life cycle of the pathogens and provide infectious organisms.

Itching, hives, and rash may appear when the organisms

first enter the skin; general aches, headache, loss of appetite, and diarrhea may follow. Later, chills, cough, abdominal pain, and other gastrointestinal symptoms may occur. Urinary symptoms, such as urinary frequency, painful urination, and bloody urine, are associated with some forms of the disease.

It is not uncommon for individuals with a mild schistosomiasis infection to be entirely free of symptoms. Apparently, rather heavy infestation is required to produce severe disease. The late complications of schistosomiasis can be quite serious, and individuals in whom infection is likely should be examined.

Schistosomiasis can be prevented by avoiding contact with infested water. However, fresh water infestation is widespread in parts of the Caribbean, South America, Africa, and Asia. Salt-water infestation does not occur. Fresh water should not be used for swimming or wading, or for drinking unless it has been boiled for ten minutes or chlorinated. Contact is most dangerous in shallow water near the banks and during bright daylight hours. Water that has been stored in clean containers for three days or more is safe for bathing. Because the infectious organisms may attach themselves to leaves, fresh vegetables, or other foods that may be contaminated by infested waters, these should not be eaten. After exposure to infested water, the skin should be rubbed vigorously with a dry towel and then with rubbing alcohol as soon as possible.

A skin infestation called swimmers itch may also be associated with schistosomal infection. Symptoms are mild rash or skin irritation and itching. This problem occurs in the Great Lakes, as well as freshwater areas of New England, Quebec, Australia, New Zealand, Germany, and Wales.

A relatively new drug called Praziquantel appears to cure all forms of schistosomiasis. Two excellent publications on schistosomiasis are available from the International Association for Medical Assistance to Travellers (see *IAMAT*).

SEAS AND SHIPS

Traveling by sea can be pleasant and relaxing, but ocean voyages may be associated with some unique medical problems. If you have little shipboard experience, a short cruise, perhaps on a smaller boat, is advisable before embarking on an extended voyage on a larger passenger cruise ship. Some persons are very prone to seasickness, and they should be aware of this fact before attempting a long cruise. Almost everyone who goes to sea will experience seasickness at some time. Be prepared. Consult the entry on *Motion Sickness*.

Another health concern for sea travel is the sanitary condition of the ship. The Communicable Disease Center (CDC) routinely inspects passenger ships docked at U.S. ports. The major purpose of these inspections is to prevent outbreaks of gastrointestinal diseases aboard ship. The CDC sets certain standards for the cleanliness of food handlers and food preparation techniques which emphasize practices for preventing food contamination, including inspection of refrigeration and water supply.

A copy of the latest inspection report for a specific passenger vessel may be obtained by writing to: Office of the Chief, Sanitation and Vector Control Activity, Quarantine Division, 1015 North America Way, Room 107, Miami, Florida 33132. A summary of the latest cruise ship sanitation inspections which lists results of inspections for all ships visiting U.S. ports is also available from this office.

Other possible medical problems could arise if there is an accident at sea. Although highly unlikely, a shipwreck could bring in addition to physical injuries, risks of drowning and exposure to cold ocean temperatures.

Learning how to swim is advisable if you plan to travel by sea or to spend any considerable amount of time around water. The ability to swim may mean the difference between death and survival in the event of an accident. Because rescue at sea generally takes some time, the ability to remain afloat may be even more critical.

Hypothermia, a severe drop in body temperature, is another hazard of accidents at sea. At water temperatures below 70°F (21°C), the body temperature will fall to below normal and will eventually decline to fatal levels. Individuals differ in their susceptibility to hypothermia, but the cooler the water, the more quickly the body temperature drops. Anyone submerged for even a few minutes in water colder than 50°F (10°C) will develop hypothermia.

In the event of a sea disaster, avoid being submerged, if possible. Wear layers of clothing that will trap air and help you to keep warm. Remain calm and follow the plan practiced during lifeboat drills. Enter the water as a last resort, and, if this become necessary, leave your clothing on and move about as little as possible. Physical activity in the water will lead to exhaustion and will cause your body temperature to fall more quickly. Stay with the other passengers in the water.

SEXUALLY-TRANSMITTED DISEASES

STD, or sexually-transmitted disease is a group of infectious disorders that may be transmitted by sexual contact. These diseases occur throughout the world in epidemic proportions. Although the likelihood of contracting STD through contact with prostitutes is high, social contacts more often spread the disease.

Symptoms of STD may vary from a single sore or a group of sores in the area of contact (genitals, lips and mouth, or rectum), to burning on urination, to a generalized rash with or without genital lesions. Many individuals with STD have no symptoms or only mild symptoms, such as penile or vaginal discharge or itching, that are dismissed as normal.

The most common sexually-transmitted diseases are gonorrhea, herpes simplex, syphilis, trichomoniasis, pediculosis (lice, crabs), venereal warts, and nonspecific urethritis or vaginitis. Other less common diseases include chancroid, lymphogranuloma venereum, granuloma inguinale, and fungal infections. A medical examination and laboratory tests are required to make a specific diagnosis and to select the proper treatment.

Prevention of STD may be accomplished by avoiding sexual relations. Condoms will offer some protection but are not infallible. The prophylactic use of antibiotics, such as high doses of ampicillin or tetracycline, immediately before or after sexual contact can offer some protection from gonorrhea and syphilis, but will not prevent herpes or some of the other sexually-transmitted diseases. Most of these diseases, with the exception of herpes simplex, can be cured with proper treatment, although gonorrhea contracted in certain areas of the world, such as large coastal cities or the Philippines, is sometimes relatively resistant to penicillin and will not respond to the usual method of treatment. Contacts and sexual partners must be treated simultaneously if reinfection is to be avoided.

The following symptoms may indicate STD: penile discharge, vaginal discharge, rectal discharge, burning on urination, a sore in the genital or rectal area, generalized rash or itching of the genital or rectal area. If a sexual contact develops a venereal disease, you must assume that you are infected and seek medical attention, even if symptoms are absent. These diseases rarely constitute medical emergencies, so there is no need to panic if you cannot obtain immediate medical care. If you suspect that you are infected with one of these diseases, refrain from sexual activity and practice good hygiene until medical care is available. Because topical home remedies will not cure sexually-transmitted diseases and may even worsen conditions, self treatment should be avoided. Some of these diseases can result in serious long-term complications or even death following weeks to years of infection, so symptoms should not be ignored, even if they disappear without treatment. Be sure to tell your doctor about your travels and your sexual contacts if there is any possibility that you may have contracted STD.

STD and certain other contagious illness are special problems for homosexuals. In addition to the usual sexually-transmitted diseases experienced by heterosexuals, homosexuals have a high incidence of hepatitis B (serum hepatitis), rectal gonorrhea, and pharyngeal gonorrhea, as well as more unusual diseases, such as acquired immune deficiency syndrome (AIDS), Kaposi's sarcoma, toxoplasmosis, and rectal herpes. Homosexuals who develop an illness while traveling should be sure to inform their doctors of their homosexual contacts, as well as of the countries in which these contacts occurred.

SMALLPOX

Smallpox was a serious infectious disease caused by a virus. However, because the disease no longer exists, there is no need for smallpox vaccinations, and most countries have discontinued routine vaccinations. International certificates of smallpox vaccination were previously required for travelers, but this is no longer the case.

STROKES

Individuals who have experienced recent strokes should probably not travel by air. Associated diseases, such as high blood pressure or heart disease, should be under reasonable control before traveling. Check with your private physician concerning your travel plans and ask for recommendations. Many stroke victims all over the world travel without undue concern. There are even special tours and trips for those with physical disabilities; check with your travel agent.

SUN EXPOSURE

Ultraviolet light causes reddening of the skin (sunburn), as well as tanning. Aging of the skin and skin cancers also result from the sun's ultraviolet light. Some individuals will have photosensitivity reactions to the sun, especially when they take certain medications (see list below). Light-skinned individuals are more sensitive to the damaging effects of the sun than are darker-skinned persons; however, anyone may become sunburned with enough exposure.

In temperate areas, most ultraviolet exposure occurs between 10:00 A.M. and 3:00 P.M. Exposure may be somewhat longer closer to the equator, and increases approximately 4% for each 1000-foot increase in altitude. Fresh snow, white surfaces, sand, and water can all reflect ultraviolet rays and thereby increase exposure. Aspirin taken before exposure to sunlight may offer some protection. A good sunscreen is recommended, especially for vulnerable areas, such as the nose, shoulders, and head.

Shade and cloud cover offer some protection from the sun, but this protection is not complete. Dry, close-knit clothing offers effective protection, but wet or loosely-knit material is much less effective. Clear water allows much of the ultraviolet light to penetrate, so being underwater does not necessarily provide protection from sun damage.

Once sunburn occurs, further exposure to the sun should be avoided. Cool compresses may be applied and analgesics, such as aspirin, may help to relieve pain. The body temperature should be taken to make sure that it is not elevated. Certain diseases, such as lupus, porphyria, solar urticaria, and some types of acne, may worsen upon exposure to sunlight.

Sunburn is exacerbated by concomitant exposure to wind, heat, moisture, and water and by the use of certain medications. The night before exposure to the sun, the skin should be hydrated with a hot shower and a sunscreen containing 5% to 10% para-minobenzoic acid, or 6% to 10% benzophenones, should be applied. Reapply the sunscreen before exposure the next day, after coming out of water and whenever there is discomfort or a change in the color of the skin is noted. Do not depend on a wet T-shirt, which offers little protection. Sunburn may be first-degree (red skin) or second-degree (blisters) and is treated like any burn.

Sunscreens are liquid preparations that block some of the damaging ultraviolet rays. The relative effectiveness is indicated by the sun protection factor or SPF. Higher SPF numbers indicate greater protection from the reddening effects of the sun. A number of different sunscreens are available and all are most effective if applied approximately one hour before exposure. They should be reapplied after bathing, sweating, or swimming. Most tanning lotions are really sunscreens and help prevent sunburn but do not really promote tanning.

Common sense is the best preventative of painful sunburn or worse. Highly sensitive individuals should always apply sunscreen and limit sun exposure, especially from midmorning until midafternoon.

Medications That Increase Sensitivity to the Sun

tetracyclines (antibiotics)
quinidine
sulfonamides (antibiotics)
phenothiazines (tranquilizers)
carbamazepine (Tegretol)
methoxsalen (Oxsoralen)
thiazides (diuretics)

Skin Contacts That Increase Sensitivity to the Sun

parsley
meadow grass
some toilet waters and perfumes
coal tar
some soaps

Sunscreens (SPF)

Aramis SPF 20 Sun Protection (20)
Clinique SPF 19 Sun Block (19)

TI Screen (15+)
Elizabeth Arden Sun Blocking Cream (15)
Eclipse, total (15)
Super Shade 15, Coppertone (15)
Bain de Soleil, Ultra Sun Block 15 (15)
PreSun 15 (15)
Block Out Cream Lotion (15)
Aramis 900 SPF 10 Sunburn Protection (10)
Estee Lauder Invisible Sun Control (10)
Advanced Sun Protection (10)
RP Paque (10)
A. Fil (8)
Bain de Soleil Sun-Filter Cream 8 (8)
Clinique 8 SPF Sun Block (8)
Maxafil (7)
Sundown Extra Protection (6)
Estee Lauder Moisturizing Sun Lotion (6)
Sundare Creamy (5)
Sea & Ski Golden Tan (4)
Coppertone Lotion (4)
PreSun 4 (4)
Bain de Soleil Moisture Tanning Face Creme 4 (4)
For Faces Only Sunscreen Coppertone 2 (2)
Bain de Soleil, Deep Tanning Oil 2 (2)
Tropic Sun Oil, Lotion (2)

SURGERY

Recent surgery is often considered a contraindication to air travel. However, medical experience in recent wars has shown that even the seriously wounded and patients who have recently undergone an operation can travel safely by air if proper facilities are available. The timing and methods of travel available to such patients depends on a number of variables, including the type of operation, the length of time since surgery, associated medical problems, and the facilities and expertise available locally. Check with your surgeon and follow his or her advice concerning travel. Ambulance companies can often assist you and act as a resource for referral to air ambulances and other specialized services. These services can be very expensive and frequently are not covered by insurance. Consider the financial aspects along with the other variables when making travel decisions.

SWIMMING

Swimming can be an enjoyable and healthy exercise, but certain basic safety rules should always be observed. Learn to swim before exposing yourself to a situation, such as fishing, boating, or traveling by water, in which the ability to swim may be essential for survival. Children should be taught to swim as soon as possible and should be accompanied by a swimmer. Never swim alone and never dive into an unknown area or into shallow water. Be especially careful when swimming in strange areas or cold water, or when medical problems exist. Know your limitations and use common sense. Do not drink alcohol or use drugs while swimming.

Chlorinated pools should be considered as the only safe areas for swimming in an area unfamiliar to you. Avoid submerging your head when swimming in waters you suspect may be contaminated. Infections of the ear, eye, or intestine may result from such contamination. Fresh water may contain organisms such as schistosomiasis or hookworm, strongyloidiasis, and cutaneous larva migrans, that may infect a swimmer standing or wading in the water.

A relatively rare form of meningitis caused by various amoebae may be contracted from swimming in still, blackish water in the United States and other countries. Diving from great heights tends to increase the probability of such infection.

Sharks. Shark attacks are uncommon but should be considered if you plan to swim in areas where dangerous sharks have been seen before. Most shark attacks occur in relatively shallow water. Experts believe that shark attacks are more likely to occur at night and in water containing blood, vomit, or excrement, as might occur when cleaning or spearing fish. When sharks are sighted, leave the water. Avoid beaches where recent shark attacks have occurred. Muddy water will hide sharks from your view but will not hide you from the sharks. Swim in clear water if possible.

If a shark should attack, stay close to your companions and swim as smoothly and quietly as possible away from the shark. Use whatever type of weapon is available to repel the shark, hitting at the eyes and gills. Keep the shark within your field of vision at all times. If a companion is attacked and needs help, it may be comforting to know that individuals who rescue shark victims are almost never attacked; rather the sharks tend to concentrate on their chosen victim. Once the bitten victim is rescued, apply direct pressure to control bleeding wounds and transport the patient to a medical facility as soon as possible.

Sharks are found in all of the seas of the world and have even been found in fresh water, for example, Lake Nicaragua and rivers. The international shark-attack files show the total number of attacks that have occurred in various areas. The following figures for U.S. shores were obtained from these files.

California	over 46	South Carolina	over 23
New Jersey	over 17	Florida	over 10
New York	8	Georgia	6
Texas	6	Massachusetts	over 4
North Carolina	2	Virginia	2
Connecticut	1	Mississippi	1

The so-called worldwide shark belt extends from a latitude of 42° south to 42° north and constitutes the area in which swimmers may encounter sharks. These waters are warm enough for bathing. Multiple shark attacks have also occurred in the waters off Puerto Rico, Central America, Africa, Mexico, India, Australia, and most other countries in this area. The swimmers most vulnerable to attack are those who swim away from the crowds, especially those who engage in spear fishing.

TYPHOID FEVER

Typhoid fever is caused by a bacterium that is introduced by ingestion of food or water contaminated by human feces. Fever, abdominal pain, headache, and general toxicity with various complications are common in untreated cases, which are often fatal. Treatment with certain antibiotics (chloramphenicol, ampicillin, trimethoprim/sulfamethox) is effective.

Typhoid fever can best be prevented by following recommendations for safe food and water (see *Foods* and *Water*). A somewhat but not completely effective vaccine is available but it does not eliminate the need for avoiding contaminated food or water. Typhoid vaccine is often recommended when traveling to endemic areas outside the United States, especially developing countries. The initial vaccine requires two doses, one week apart, and boosters must be given yearly. Most of the 500 cases of typhoid that occur each year in the U.S. affect travelers who have been to Mexico or India, or some endemic area of Asia, Africa, or the Far East.

TYPHUS

Typhus is an infectious disease caused by a tiny organism related to the one responsible for Rocky Mountain spotted fever. The symptoms of the fully developed disease include chills, fever, and severe headache, as well as a generalized rash that appears a few days later. The infection is found all over the world and is transmitted when infected flea or louse feces enters broken skin.

Good hygiene is effective in preventing typhus, and few travelers are exposed to fleas or lice these days. Typhus is easily treated with available antibiotics (tetracycline or chloramphenicol). A vaccine is available outside the U.S. but is not recommended because the risk of infection is small.

VACCINES AND INOCULATIONS

The immunizations advised for any specific trip will depend on many factors, including your own history of illness and immunization, the places you intend to visit, the advice of your personal physician, and your own opinion. Because recommendations and travel requirements are constantly changing, you or your physician should obtain updated information from the U.S. Public Health Service. The publications most useful are *Health Information for International Travel*, and the *Morbidity and Mortality Weekly Report*, and which may be requested from the Superintendent of Documents, U.S. Government Printing Office, Washington, DC 20402.

Each immunization, like any other medication, has specific

contraindications, that is, situations in which they should not be administered. For example, live vaccines* should not be given to certain immuno-suppressed persons such as those who have leukemia or who are receiving certain drugs. When a contraindicated vaccine is required by law, you may obtain a letter from your physician explaining the situation and outlining the medical reasons why you have not received a specific vaccine.

Certain vaccines, such as typhoid, plague, and cholera vaccines, may cause uncomfortable side effects and should not be given at the same time. Many other vaccines may be given simultaneously at different sites. Your vaccines should be timed so that any side effects have resolved by the time you begin your trip. Also, because gamma globulin may interfere with the development of immunity, gamma globulin should not be given until at least ten days after administration of the last vaccine needed.

The following vaccines are of greatest interest to the traveler.

Cholera vaccine is a killed* vaccine. Some countries require a single dose no longer than six months before entering that country from an infected area. Because the risk of contracting cholera is usually very low, cholera vaccine is not recommended unless you are traveling to a country where it is required for entry. Some vaccinated individuals experience a few days of local pain, swelling or general fever, malaise, and headache. Pregnant women should not receive cholera vaccine.

Infectious Hepatitis immunoglobulin (gamma globulin) will prevent infectious hepatitis (hepatitis A) if given before exposure. The 2-ml dose should be given intramuscularly shortly before departing but at least ten days after the last of any vaccine taken. This dose will offer protection for up to three months. If longer protection is desired, a dose of 5 ml may be given. Immunoglobulin is recommended for travelers to all areas with the exception of the United States and Canada. Risks are highest

*A live vaccine is an actual organism that can multiply and grow but does not cause disease in humans. The human body produces antibodies in reaction to these organisms, making the vaccinated person immune. Immunity is long-lived and may even be permanent.

*A killed vaccine is not infectious. It poses no danger to even immuno-suppressed individuals. The body produces antibodies to a killed vaccine to produce an immunity to the disease which is not permanent and requires "booster" shots.

in developing and tropical countries and for travelers who bypass the usual tourist routes. These risks increase in individuals who stay for more than three months in areas with questionable public health practices. For short-term (less than three months) travel, the recommended dose in children is 0.5 ml for those under 50 pounds, and 1 ml for children between 50 and 100 pounds. For more extended travel, doses of 1 ml and 2.5 ml, respectively, are recommended. Children over 100 pounds should receive adult doses.

Measles vaccine is a live vaccine recommended for all travelers born after 1956 with no documented history of measles infection or vaccination. No country requires this vaccine for entry. Pregnant women, individuals with congenital immunologic deficiencies, leukemia, lymphoma, or generalized cancers, and those receiving immunosuppressive drugs or radiation therapy should not receive measles vaccine.

Plague vaccine is a killed vaccine that is frequently associated with side effects. It is recommended only for travelers who may come in contact with wild rodents, such as rats, rabbits, and prairie dogs, or fleas in endemic areas, which include the southwestern United States, Lao People's Democratic Republic (Laos), Vietnam, Democratic Kompuc MA (Cambodia), and other areas in Africa, Asia, and South America. No country requires this vaccine for entry. Full immunization takes a minimum of three doses given over an eight-week period.

Polio vaccine is recommended for all travelers, especially for those visiting developing or tropical countries, both live and killed vaccines are available. Persons who have been immunized previously should receive one dose of live trivalent oral polio vaccine. Previously unimmunized individuals should receive a full series, before traveling, preferably of live trivalent oral vaccine. No country requires polio vaccine for entry. Immuno-compromised persons and their families should receive inactivated polio vaccine. The minimal time needed for full primary vaccination is ten months. Shorter schedules may provide some protection in four to eight weeks.

Rabies vaccine is an inactivated viral vaccine and is recommended for travelers who may contact rabid animals or who plan long visits to an area where rabies is a constant threat. Countries in which human rabies occur relatively frequently include Mexico and India

Those who expect to visit caves which have infected bats or who plan to handle potentially infected animals, such as bats, skunks, foxes, dogs, raccoons, and cats, in endemic areas should have a full series with the diploid-cell rabies vaccine. No country requires rabies vaccine for entry.

Smallpox vaccine is a live virus vaccine that is no longer recommended for travel. Although smallpox has been eradicated, a few countries require an International Certificate of Vaccination against smallpox. These countries (Chad, Democratic Kompuc MA) will accept a written statement from a physician that vaccination is medically contraindicated.

Tetanus/diphtheria is an inactivated toxin vaccine. Everyone should receive a primary series. Booster doses should be given every ten years. No country requires this vaccine for entry.

Typhoid vaccine is a killed bacterial vaccine. Administration of this vaccine is often associated with side effects, such as pain at the injection site, fever, headache, and malaise. Although no country requires the typhoid vaccine for entry, all travelers to rural tropical areas should receive this vaccine every three years.

Typhus vaccine is a killed vaccine. It is not generally recommended for travelers and is no longer manufactured in the United States.

Yellow Fever vaccine is a live virus recommended for travelers to areas where yellow fever is endemic. Some countries require a yellow fever certificate for entry if you have traveled through an infected area or are entering the country from an endemic zone. Endemic areas are those countries with a latitude between 15° north and 15° south and include African countries, Panama, Venezuela, Surinam, Guyana, French Guiana, Columbia, Brazil, Peru, Bolivia, Ecuador, and the Caribbean nations.

Yellow fever vaccine is the only vaccine that cannot be obtained from your own physician. It must be administered at a designated Yellow Fever Vaccination Center. Your local health department can tell you the location of centers in your area. Once you have received the vaccine, it is effective for ten years. Pregnant women traveling to high-risk areas should be vaccinated if they cannot avoid exposure to yellow fever. However, it is preferable to avoid both the vaccine and yellow fever exposure during pregnancy. Individuals with leukemia, lymphoma, or generalized cancer and those being treated with corticosteroid or anticancer drugs, such as alkylating agents and antimetabolites, or radiation should not receive this vaccine.

VIRAL HEMORRHAGIC FEVER (VHF)

The name viral hemorrhagic fever (VHF) is derived from the bleeding, usually in the skin and bowel, that occurs in severe cases. Although this group of diseases rarely afflicts travelers, anyone traveling to Africa, Asia, or Eastern Europe may be exposed to one of these viral illnesses. Each of these infections is caused by a specific virus endemic to a particular area, as shown in the following chart:

	Lassa Fever	Efala Hemorrhagic Fever	Marburg Virus Disease	Crimean-Campo Hemorrhagic Fever
Endemic area	W. Africa, from Guiana to Central Africa	E. Africa, Zaire, Sudan, Central Africa, Rep. of Kenya	E. Africa, S. Africa	Asia, Africa, Eastern Europe

Symptoms of infection are similar and closely resemble those of other infections characterized by fever, sore throat, headache, myalgia, cough, and gastrointestinal discomfort with nausea, vomiting, and diarrhea. Patients with mild cases may have only a few symptoms: a rash is not infrequent. Patients with severe cases will have bleeding from the bowel with bloody diarrhea and/or vomiting. Bruises on the skin may indicate bleeding into the skin. Bleeding can result in shock and death. Abdominal and/or chest pains are not uncommon and may be severe.

Obviously there are many more common diseases with similar symptoms. Malaria, typhoid fever, menigococcal infection, leptospirosis, and other viral infections (arbovirus enterovirus) are much more common than VHF.

Prevention is the only method of effectively dealing with VHF; there is no specific treatment. No vaccines are available. Avoidance of animals and persons who are obviously ill is probably the most reasonable approach to prevention. Because tick bites may also result in infection, antitick measures are also recommended.

Anyone who is suspected of having VHF should be transported to a modern medical facility and placed in isolation. Supportive treatment may reduce mortality, and isolation will prevent the spread of infection. Some epidemics of VHF have been associated with a high mortality rate.

WATER, DON'T DRINK THE...

Contaminated water is another potential cause of illness while traveling. Chlorination of drinking water will prevent most waterborne viral and bacterial diseases. Water in many hotels in large cities is chlorinated. Chlorination, however, does not reliably kill certain parasites, such as *Giardia* and amoeba.

Boiling water for ten minutes and then allowing it to cool is another means of purification. Do not, however, add ice once the water has been boiled. Another method of water treatment is the use of tincture of iodine (25%). Five drops should be added to each quart or liter of clear water, and the treated water should then be allowed to stand for 30 minutes before it is used. If the water is cold or cloudy, ten drops of tincture of iodine should be used, and the water should be allowed to stand for five hours or more. Commercial disinfectant tablets are also available. Directions for use are supplied with these tablets.

You can chlorinate your own water with liquid chlorine laundry bleach, which is available at grocery stores. The percent of chlorine should be stated on the bottle. Use ten drops of bleach per quart or liter of clear water if the chlorine concentration is 1%, use two drops if it is 4% to 6%, use one drop if it is between 7% and 10%. If the water is cold or cloudy, use twice the number of drops recommended for clear water. Allow clear water to stand for thirty minutes before using it and allow cold or cloudy water to stand for five hours or more.

A slight chlorine odor should be detectable after the water has been allowed to stand. Remember, chlorination kills only bacteria and viruses, not parasites.

A number of illnesses may be transmitted by drinking water. Typhoid fever, paratyphoid, cholera, Campylobacter infections, shigellosis, tularemia and *Escherichia coli* infections are among the waterborne bacterial diseases. Viruses such as the Norwalk agent, polio, and hepatitis viruses, may also be waterborne. Amoeba, *Giardia*, and certain parasitic worms that may also be found in water are not affected by chlorination, although there are other methods of purification for eliminating these organisms. Noninfectious contaminants, such as radioactive material, pesticides, and other chemical contaminants, such as lead, nitrates and fluorides, may cause illness, but the usual traveler is not likely to encounter such substances.

YELLOW FEVER

Yellow fever is a viral disease transmitted to humans by mosquitoes. It is presently confined to tropical and subtropical areas of the world. The illness can vary from a mild fever with headache to a severe disease associated with bleeding, coma, and death. Occasionally, the severely ill patient is obviously yellow (jaundiced), thus accounting for the name.

Yellow fever vaccine is effective in preventing illness and is advised for those entering infected areas. Some countries require this vaccine for anyone entering from an infected area.

ENDEMIC AREAS FOR YELLOW FEVER

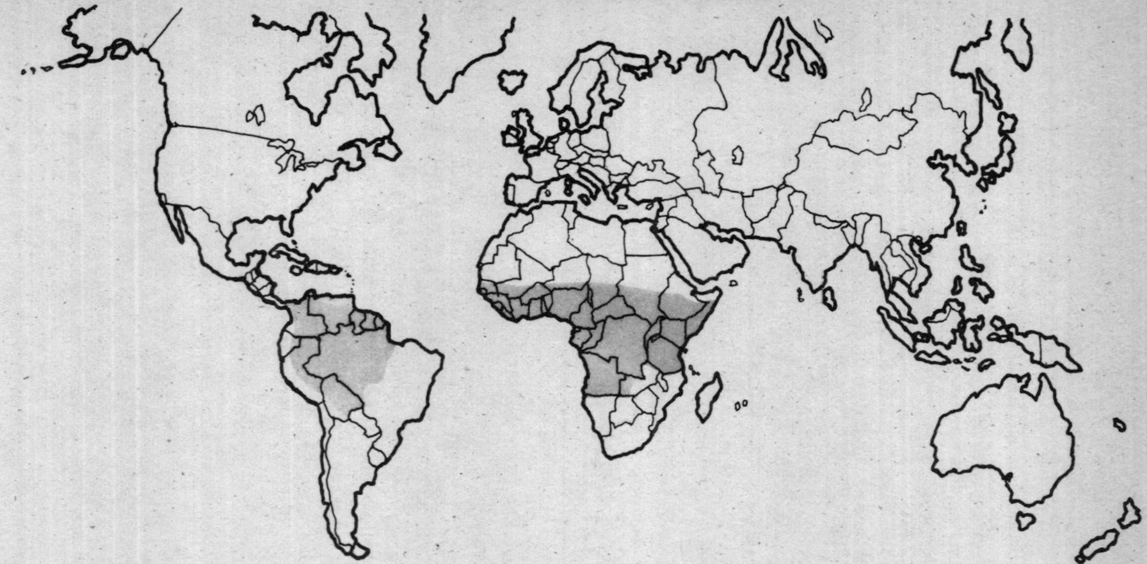

A Worldwide Directory of Required and Recommended Immunizations and Traveler's Cautions

If you are considering travel to a foreign country, consult this list to determine which immunizations you need, what conditions to be aware of, and whether you can locate an IAMAT English-speaking physician at that locale.

AFGHANISTAN

No IAMAT doctor; water, milk products, and cold food unsafe

Required

Yellow Fever vaccine if in infected country during preceding 14 days.

Risks

Malaria, all areas May–Nov. under 2000 meters (6600 ft.) recommend chloroquine prophylaxis

Infectious hepatitis, recommend 2 cc gamma globulin

Typhus, recommend vaccine if outside tourist areas or working there

Polio, Diphtheria, Tetanus, recommend updating vaccine

ALBANIA

No IAMAT doctor; water probably safe but not recommended; milk and food safe

Required

Cholera vaccine (persons over 6 mos. old), *Yellow fever vaccine* (persons over one year old) if from infected area preceding 14 days

Risks

Typhoid, vaccine recommended if work there or outside tourist areas

Diphtheria, Tetanus, Polio, recommend updating vaccine

ALGERIA

IAMAT doctor available; water, milk products, and cold food unsafe

Required

Yellow Fever vaccine (over age one) if from infected area preceding 14 days

Risks

Malaria, in rural areas of Ourargla, Wilaya if departure May–Nov. recommend chloroquine prophylaxis

Infectious hepatitis, recommend 2 cc gamma globulin

Thyphoid, vaccine recommended if work there or outside tourist areas

Diphtheria, Tetanus, Polio, recommend updating vaccines

AMERICAN SAMOA (Pago Pago)

IAMAT doctor available; water probably safe but not recommended; milk products and food safe

Required

Yellow fever vaccine (those over age one) if from infected area preceding 14 days

Risks

Diphtheria, Tetanus, Polio, recommend updating vaccines

Dingue fever, use mosquito nets and/or screens, mosquito repellents

ANDORRA

No IAMAT doctor available; water probably safe but not recommended; milk products and food safe

Required

None

Risks

No significant, recommend updating *Diphtheria, Tetanus*, and *Polio* vaccines

ANGOLA

IAMAT doctor available in Luanda; water, milk products, and cold food unsafe

Required

Cholera and *Yellow fever vaccines* (over age one) if from infected area preceding 14 days

Risks

Yellow fever, vaccine recommended

Infectious hepatitis, recommend 2 cc gamma globulin

Typhoid, recommend vaccine

Polio, Diphtheria, Tetanus, recommend updating vaccines

ANTIGUA

No IAMAT doctor available; water, milk products, and food safe

Required

Yellow fever vaccine (over age one) if from infected area

Risks

No significant, recommend updating *Diphtheria, Tetanus* and *Polio* vaccines

ARGENTINA

IAMAT doctors available, water probably safe but not recommended; milk products and food safe

Required

None

Risks

Infectious hepatitis, recommend 2 cc gamma globulin

Typhoid fever, vaccine recommended for workers or outside tourist areas

Diphtheria, Tetanus, Polio, vaccine update recommended

AUSTRALIA

IAMAT doctors available; water, milk products, and food safe

Required

Yellow fever vaccine required (over age one) if from infected country preceding 14 days

Risks

Infectious hepatitis, recommended 2 cc gamma globulin

Dingue, along coast from Cornavon to Port Darwin to Townsville and occasionally northern New South Wales, recommend mosquito repellent

Diphtheria, Tetanus, Polio, recommend updating vaccine

Lyme arthritis, avoid ticks

AUSTRIA

No IAMAT doctors available; water probably safe but not recommended, milk products and food safe

Required

None

Risks

None, recommend updating *Diphtheria, Tetanus* and *Polio* vaccines

AZORES

No IAMAT doctor; water probably safe but not recommended; milk products and food safe

Required

Yellow fever vaccine (over age one) if from infected area previous 14 days

Risks

None, recommend updating *Diphtheria, Tetanus*, and *Polio* vaccines

BAHAMAS

IAMAT doctor available; water, milk products, and cold food unsafe

Required

Yellow fever vaccine (over age one) if from infected area preceding 14 days

Risks

None, recommend updating *Diphtheria* and *Tetanus* vaccines

BAHRAIN

No IAMAT doctor; water, milk products, and cold food unsafe

Required

Yellow fever vaccine (over age one) if from infected country previous 14 days

Risks

Infectious hepatitis, recommend 2 cc gamma globulin

Typhoid fever, recommend vaccine

Diphtheria, Tetanus, Polio, update vaccines

Malaria, all areas (urban & rural) all year, recommend chloroquine prophylaxis

BANGLADESH

IAMAT doctor available in Dacca; water, milk products, and cold food unsafe

Required

Yellow fever vaccine required if in infected area previous 14 days (including many African & South American countries)

Risks

Cholera, consider vaccine, full food and drink precautions

Infectious hepatitis, recommend 2 cc gamma globulin

Rabies, pre-exposure vaccine if animal exposure likely, avoid animals, post-exposure treatment after any animal bite

Typhoid, vaccine recommended, full food and drink precautions

Diphtheria, Polio, Tetanus, recommend update vaccine

Malaria, including resistant falciparum, recommend chloroquine and Fansidar prophylaxis

Yellow fever, vaccination recommended

BARBADOS

No IAMAT doctor available; water, milk and food safe

Required

Yellow fever vaccine (over age one) if in infected area previous 14 days

Risks

None, recommend updating *Diphtheria*, *Tetanus* and *Polio* vaccines

BELGIUM

IAMAT doctor available; water, milk products, food safe

Required

None

Risks

None, recommend updating *Diphtheria*, *Polio* and *Tetanus* vaccines

BELIZE (formerly British Honduras)

No IAMAT doctor; water, milk products, and cold food unsafe

Required

Yellow fever vaccine (over age one) if from infected area previous 14 days

Risks

Infectious hepatitis, recommend 2 cc gamma globulin

Typhoid, recommend vaccine if outside the usual tourist areas

Diphtheria, Polio, Tetanus, recommend updating vaccines

Malaria, in all rural areas except Gelize Dist., year round below 1320 ft. (400 m), recommend chloroquine prophylaxis

Dingue, recommend mosquito repellent

BENIN

No IAMAT doctor; water unsafe; milk may be unsafe because of poor refrigeration; other milk products safe; cold food unsafe

Required

Yellow fever vaccine (over age one)

Risks

Yellow fever, vaccination recommended

Infectious hepatitis, recommend 2 cc gamma globulin

Typhoid, vaccination recommended

Diphtheria, Polio, Tetanus, vaccination recommended

Malaria, in all areas, year-round

Cholera, avoid water and cold food

BERMUDA

No IAMAT doctor; water, milk, and food are safe

Required

None

Risks

None, recommend *Diphtheria*, *Polio* and *Tetanus* vaccines

BHUTAN

No IAMAT doctor; water, milk and cold food unsafe

Required

None

Risks

Infectious hepatitis, recommend 2 cc gamma globulin

Typhus, louseborn, vaccine recommended

Typhoid, vaccine recommended

Diphtheria, Tetanus, Polio, vaccines recommended

Malaria, all rural areas (except Chirang, Sanchi) all year below 5280 ft. (1600 m), recommend chloroquine prophylaxis

BOLIVIA

IAMAT doctor available; water, milk products, and cold food unsafe

Required

Yellow fever vaccine if from infected area previous 14 days and for all travelers to Santa Cruz de la Sierra

Risks

Yellow fever, vaccination strongly recommended

Infectious hepatitis, recommend 2 cc gamma globulin

Malaria, year-round in rural areas below 6600 ft. (2000 m) except for La Paz, Oruro, Potosī Province, recommend chloroquine prophylaxis

Plague, vaccine recommended for those exposed to wild rodents; those not vaccinated, may take prophylactic sulfonamides daily

Typhus, vaccination recommended, good personal hygiene important

Typhoid, vaccination recommended if outside tourist areas

Diphtheria, Tetanus, Polio, vaccination recommended.

BOTSWANA

IAMAT doctor available; water, milk products, and cold food unsafe in some areas

Required

Yellow fever vaccine (over age one) if from infected area previous 14 days

Risks

Infectious hepatitis, recommend 2 cc gamma globulin

Typhus, vaccine recommended if outside tourist area

Typhoid, vaccine recommended

Diphtheria, Polio, Tetanus, vaccine recommended

Malaria, northern part from Nov.–May in both urban and rural areas, chloroquine prophylaxis recommended

BRAZIL

IAMAT doctors available; water, milk products and cold food unsafe

Required

Yellow fever vaccine (over age one) if in infected area previous 14 days; *polio vaccine* required for children three mos. to 6 years of age

Risks

Yellow fever, vaccine recommended for those outside cities

Infectious hepatitis, recommend 2 cc gamma globulin

Plague, recommend vaccination for those exposed to wild rodents, those not vaccinated may take prophylactic sulfonamides daily

Typhoid, recommend vaccination

Diphtheria, Polio, Tetanus, recommend vaccination

Malaria, many areas both rural and urban (along Amazon River) year-round below 3000 ft. (900 m); some chloroquine resistant falciparum in interior coastal area north of Rio de Janeiro, recommend chloroquine prophylaxis, also Fansidar.

BRUNEI

No IAMAT doctor available; water, milk products, and cold food unsafe

Required

Cholera and *Yellow fever vaccines* (over age one) if in infected country previous 14 days

Risks

Infectious hepatitis, recommend 2 cc gamma globulin

Typhoid, recommend vaccination

Diphtheria, Polio, Tetanus, vaccine recommended

BULGARIA

No IAMAT doctor; water probably safe but not recommended; milk products and food safe

Required

None

Risks

None, recommend updating *Diphtheria, Polio* and *Tetanus* vaccines

BURKINA FASO (Formerly Upper Volta)

No IAMAT doctor available; water, milk products, and cold food unsafe

Required

Yellow fever vaccine for all travelers over age one

Risks

Infectious Hepatitis, recommend 2 cc gamma globulin

Rabies, recommend pre-exposure vaccine, avoid mammals

Typhoid, recommend vaccine

Diphtheria, Polio, Tetanus, recommend updating vaccines

Malaria, in all areas, year-round, recommend chloroquine prophylaxis

BURMA

IAMAT doctor available; water, milk products, and cold food unsafe

Required

Cholera vaccine; Yellow fever vaccine if from infected area previous 14 days or from certain African, Central American and South American countries

Risks

Cholera, vaccine recommended if working in primitive areas and those with low acid in stomach (e.g., on antacids, post-ulcer surgery, marijuana smokers)

Infectious hepatitis, recommend 2 cc gamma globulin

Plague, recommend vaccination for those exposed to wild rodents, sulfonamide prophylaxis daily can offer protection in unvaccinated

Rabies, recommend vaccine for those on working assignments, avoid mammals, if bitten obtain postexposure treatment

Typhus, recommend vaccine if outside tourist areas

Typhoid, recommend vaccination

Diphtheria, Polio, Tetanus, recommend vaccination

Dengue, anti-mosquito measures from dusk to dawn, repellent, screening, nets

Malaria, from April–Dec., areas under 3300 ft. (1000 m), some chloroquine resistant, use chloroquine and Fansidar prophylaxis

BURUNDI

No IAMAT doctor; water, milk products, and cold food unsafe

Required

Yellow fever vaccine (over age one) if from infected area previous 14 days or from certain African, South American and Central American countries

Risks

Cholera, recommend vaccine for those in primitive areas and those with low stomach acid (on antacid, postoperative ulcer surgery, marijuana smokers)

Yellow Fever, recommend vaccination

Infectious hepatitis, recommend 2 cc gamma globulin

Typhus, recommend vaccine for those outside usual tourist area

Typhoid, recommend vaccination

Diphtheria, Polio, Tetanus, recommend vaccination

Malaria, in all areas, year-round, recommend chloroquine prophylaxis

CAMEROON, UNITED REPUBLIC OF

IAMAT doctor available; water, milk products, and cold food unsafe

Required

Yellow fever vaccine for all over age one

Risks

Cholera, recommend vaccine for those in primitive areas and those with low stomach acid (on antacids, previous ulcer surgery, marijuana smokers)

Infectious hepatitis, recommend 2 cc gamma globulin

Typhus, recommend good hygiene, vaccine for those outside usual tourist areas

Typhoid, recommend vaccine

Diphtheria, Polio, Tetanus, recommend vaccine

Malaria, in all areas, year-round, recommend chloroquine prophylaxis

CANADA

IAMAT doctors available; water, milk products, and food safe

Required

None

Risks

None, recommend *Diphtheria, Polio* and *Tetanus* vaccines

CANARY ISLANDS

IAMAT doctor available; water probably safe but not recommended; milk products and food safe

Required

None

Risks

None, recommend updating *Diphtheria, Polio* and *Tetanus* vaccines

CAPE VERDE

No IAMAT doctor available; water, milk products and cold food unsafe

Required

Cholera vaccine and *Yellow fever vaccine* (over age one) if from infected area previous 14 days, no certificate required if arriving in Boa Vista, Maio, Sal, Santiago and São Vicente

Risks

Yellow fever, recommend vaccination

Infectious hepatitis, recommend 2 cc gamma globulin

Typhoid, recommend vaccination

Diphtheria, Polio, Tetanus, recommend updating vaccines

Malaria, in rural areas of Cancelko de Santa Cruz, recommend chloroquine prophylaxis

CAYMAN ISLANDS

No IAMAT doctor available; water probably safe but not recommended; milk products and food safe

Required

None

Risks

None, recommend updating *Diphtheria, Polio* and *Tetanus* vaccines

CENTRAL AFRICAN REPUBLIC

IAMAT doctor available; water, milk, and water probably unsafe

Required

Yellow fever vaccine (all over age one)

Risks

Infectious hepatitis, recommend 2 cc of gamma globulin

Rabies, recommend pre-exposure vaccine if exposed to mammals likely, avoid dogs, cats and other mammals

Typhoid, recommend vaccination

Diphtheria, Polio, Tetanus, recommend updating vaccines

Malaria, in all areas year-round, recommend chloroquine prophylaxis

CHAD

IAMAT doctor available; water, milk products, and cold food unsafe

Required

Smallpox vaccine (over age one), recommend *not* getting vaccinated; obtain letter from doctor explaining not vaccinated for "health reasons," vaccination contraindicated

Risks

Cholera, recommend vaccination for those in rural areas and those with low stomach acid (on antacids, previous ulcer surgery, marijuana smokers)

Yellow fever, recommend vaccination for those over age one

Infectious hepatitis, recommend 2 cc of gamma globulin

Rabies, recommend pre-exposure vaccine if exposed to mammals likely, avoid dogs, cats and other mammals

Typhus, recommend vaccine if traveling outside usual tourist areas

Typhoid, recommend vaccination

Diphtheria, Polio, Tetanus, recommend updating vaccines

Malaria, all areas, July–Nov., recommend chloroquine prophylaxis

CHILE

IAMAT doctor available; water frequently unsafe and not recommended; milk products and cold food unsafe

Required

None

Risks

Infection hepatitis, recommend 2 cc gamma globulin

Typhoid, recommend vaccination

Diphtheria, Polio, Tetanus, recommend updating vaccines

CHINA, PEOPLE'S REPUBLIC OF

No IAMAT doctor available; water, milk products and cold food unsafe

Required

Yellow fever vaccine if from infected country previous 14 days

Risks

Infectious hepatitis, recommend 2 cc gamma globulin

Plague, recommend vaccine if exposure to wild rodents likely, sulfa prophylaxis if in areas with plague

Typhoid, recommend vaccine

Dengue, in some areas, apply anti-mosquito measures dusk to dawn

Diphtheria, Polio, Tetanus, recommend updating vaccines

Malaria, in some areas, primarily outside usual tourist areas, some chloroquine-resistant falciparum; at risk June–Oct. north of 33° N; May–Dec. 25° N year-round; south of 25° N, recommend chloroquine and Fansidar prophylaxis

CHINA (TAIWAN)

IAMAT doctor available; water, milk products and cold food unsafe

Required

Cholera vaccine (over age one) if from infected country last 14 days

Risks

Infectious hepatitis, recommend 2 cc of gamma globulin

Typhoid, recommend vaccine if traveling outside usual tourist areas

Diphtheria, Polio, Tetanus, recommend updating vaccines

Dengue, in some areas, apply anti-mosquito measures dusk to dawn

Malaria, primarily outside tourist areas, year-round, recommend chloroquine and Fansidar prophylaxis

CHRISTMAS ISLANDS

No IAMAT doctor available; water, milk products and food probably safe; check locally before consumption

Required

Yellow fever vaccine if from infected country last 14 days or if from many countries of Africa, Central and South America

Risks

Diphtheria, Polio, Tetanus, recommend updating vaccines

COLOMBIA

IAMAT doctor available; water, milk products, and cold food unsafe

Required

None

Risks

Yellow Fever, vaccine recommended

Infectious hepatitis, recommend 2 cc gamma globulin

Typhoid, recommend vaccine

Diphtheria, Polio, Tetanus, recommend updating vaccines

Malaria, in all rural areas, year-round under 2640 ft. (800 m), recommend chloroquine and Fansidar prophylaxis

COMOROS

No IAMAT doctor available; water, milk products, and cold food unsafe

Required

None

Risks

Infectious hepatitis, recommend 2 cc gamma globulin

Typhoid, recommend vaccine

Diphtheria, Polio, Tetanus, recommend updating vaccines

Malaria, all areas, year-round, recommend chloroquine prophylaxis

CONGO, PEOPLE'S REPUBLIC OF

IAMAT doctor available; water, milk products and food unsafe

Required

Yellow fever vaccine (over age one) except those from noninfected area and staying less than two weeks

Risks

Cholera, recommend vaccine for those living under inadequate sanitary conditions and those with low stomach acid (on antacids, previous ulcer surgery, marijuana smokers)

Infectious hepatitis, recommend 2 cc gamma globulin

Typhus, avoid lice, recommend vaccine for those in interior

Typhoid, recommend vaccine

Diphtheria, Polio, Tetanus, recommend updating vaccine

Malaria, recommend chloroquine prophylaxis

COOK ISLANDS

No IAMAT doctor available; water safe but may cause some diarrhea initially; milk products and food safe

Required

None

Risks

Dengue, apply anti-mosquito measures from dusk to dawn

Diphtheria, Polio, Tetanus, recommend updating vaccines

COSTA RICA

No IAMAT doctor; water, milk products, and food unsafe

Required

None

Risks

Infectious hepatitis, recommend 2 cc gamma globulin

Typhoid, recommend vaccine if outside usual tourist area

Diphtheria, Polio, Tetanus, recommend updating vaccines

CUBA

No IAMAT doctor available; water, milk products, and cold food unsafe

Required

Yellow fever vaccine if from infected area previous 14 days or endemic areas (Equatorial Africa, Central and South America)

Risks

Infectious hepatitis, recommend 2 cc of gamma globulin

Typhoid, recommend vaccine if outside usual tourist area

Dengue, anti-mosquito measures from dusk to dawn

Diphtheria, Polio, Tetanus, recommend updating vaccine

CYPRUS

IAMAT doctor available; water probably safe but not recommended; milk products and food safe

Required

None

Risks

Infectious hepatitis, recommend 2 cc gamma globulin

Typhoid, recommend vaccine

Dengue, recommend anti-mosquito measures dusk to dawn

Diphtheria, Polio, Tetanus, recommend updating vaccines

CZECHOSLOVAKIA

No IAMAT doctor available; water probably safe but not recommended; milk products and food safe

Required

None

Risks

Diphtheria, Polio, Tetanus, recommend updating vaccines

DENMARK

IAMAT doctor available; water, milk products, and food safe

Required

None

Risks

Diphtheria, Polio, Tetanus, recommend updating vaccines

DJIBOUTI

No IAMAT doctor available; water probably safe but not recommended; milk products and cold food unsafe

Required

Yellow fever vaccine (over age one) if from infected country previous 14 days

Risks

Infectious hepatitis, recommend 2 cc gamma globulin

Typhoid, recommend vaccine if outside usual tourist areas

Diphtheria, Polio, Tetanus, recommend updating vaccine

Malaria, all areas, recommend chloroquine prophylaxis

DOMINICA

No IAMAT doctor available; water probably safe but not recommended; milk products and food safe

Required

Yellow fever vaccine (over age one) if in infected country previous 14 days

Risks

Diphtheria, Polio, Tetanus, recommend updating vaccine

Dengue, recommend anti-mosquito measures dusk to dawn

DOMINICAN REPUBLIC

IAMAT doctor available; water, milk products, and cold food unsafe

Required

Cholera and *Yellow fever vaccines* if in infected country previous 14 days

Risks

Infectious hepatitis, recommend 2 cc of gamma globulin

Typhoid, recommend vaccine if outside usual tourist area

Diphtheria, Polio, Tetanus, recommend updating vaccines

Malaria, rural areas under 1200 ft. (400 m), especially bordering on Haiti year-round, recommend chloroquine prophylaxis

Dengue, recommend anti-mosquito measures dusk to dawn

ECUADOR

IAMAT doctor available; water, milk products, and cold food unsafe

Required

Yellow fever vaccine if in infected area previous 14 days

Risks

Yellow fever, recommend vaccine

Infectious hepatitis, recommend 2 cc gamma globulin

Typhoid, recommend vaccine

Diphtheria, Polio, Tetanus, recommend updating vaccines

Malaria, year-round under 3300 ft. (1500 m), recommend chloroquine and Fansidar prophylaxis

EGYPT

IAMAT doctor available; water probably safe but not recommended; milk products other than powdered or evaporated milk unsafe; cold food unsafe

Required

Cholera vaccine over age one if in infected area previous 14 days
Yellow fever vaccine over age one if from Africa, Central or South American countries or other infected country previous 14 days

Risks

Infectious hepatitis, recommend 2 cc gamma globulin

Rabies, recommend pre-exposure rabies vaccine, avoid mammals

Typhoid, recommend vaccine

Diphtheria, Polio, Tetanus, recommend updating vaccine

Malaria, in rural areas, Nile delta and Oases El Fai Yum and other areas June–Oct., recommend chloroquine prophylaxis

EL SALVADOR

IAMAT doctor available; water, milk products, and cold food unsafe

Required

Yellow fever vaccine (over 6 mos. old) if in infected area last 14 days

Risks

Infectious hepatitis, recommend 2 cc gamma globulin

Typhoid, recommend vaccine

Diphtheria, Polio, Tetanus, recommend updating vaccines

Malaria, in rural areas, year-round under 3300 ft. (1000m), recommend chloroquine prophylaxis

Dengue, recommend anti-mosquito measures dusk to dawn

EQUATORIAL GUINEA

No IAMAT doctor available; water, milk products, and cold food unsafe

Required

Yellow fever vaccine for all travelers

Risks

Yellow fever, recommend vaccine

Infectious hepatitis, recommend 2 cc gamma globulin

Typhoid, recommend vaccine

Diphtheria, Polio, Tetanus, recommend updating vaccines

Malaria, all areas year-round, recommend chloroquine-prophylaxis

ETHIOPIA

No IAMAT doctor available; water, milk products, and cold food unsafe

Required

Yellow fever vaccine for all travelers

Risks

Yellow Fever, recommend vaccine

Infectious hepatitis, recommend 2 cc gamma globulin

Rabies, recommend pre-exposure vaccine for anyone exposed to mammals, avoid contact with mammals

Typhus, recommend vaccine

Typhoid, recommend vaccine

Diphtheria, Polio, Tetanus, recommend updating vaccines

Malaria, recommend chloroquine prophylaxis

FAEROE ISLANDS

No IAMAT doctor available; water, milk products, and food safe

Required

None

Risks

None, recommend updating *Diphtheria*, *Polio* and *Tetanus* vaccines

FALKLAND ISLANDS

No IAMAT doctor available; water, milk products, and food safe

Required

None

Risks

None, recommend updating *Diphtheria*, *Polio* and *Tetanus* vaccines

FIJI

No IAMAT doctor available; water probably safe but not recommended; milk products and food safe

Required

Cholera and *Yellow fever* vaccines (over age one) if in infected area previous 14 days

Risks

Dengue, recommend anti-mosquito measures dusk to dawn

Diphtheria, Polio, Tetanus, recommend updating vaccines

FINLAND

IAMAT doctor available; water, milk products, and food safe

Required

None

Risks

None, recommend updating *Diphtheria*, *Polio* and *Tetanus* vaccines

FRANCE

IAMAT doctor available; water safe but not recommended, milk products and food safe

Required

None

Risks

None, recommend updating *Diphtheria*, *Polio* and *Tetanus* vaccines

GABON

IAMAT doctor available; water, milk products, and cold food unsafe

Required

Yellow fever vaccine (over age one) if in infected area previous 14 days

Risks

Yellow fever, recommend vaccine

Infectious hepatitis, recommend 2 cc gamma globulin

Typhoid, recommend vaccine

Diphteria, Polio, Tetanus, recommend updating vaccines

Malaria, all areas, year-round under 3300 ft. (1000 m), recommend chloroquine prophylaxis

GAMBIA

No IAMAT doctor available; water, milk products, and food unsafe

Required

Yellow fever vaccine for all travelers over age one

Risks

Infectious hepatitis, recommend 2 cc gamma globulin

Typhoid, recommend vaccine

Diphtheria, Polio, Tetanus, recommend updating vaccines

Malaria, in all areas, year-round, recommend chloroquine prophylaxis

GERMAN DEMOCRATIC REPUBLIC

No IAMAT doctor available; See Federal Republic of Germany (below)

GERMANY, FEDERAL REPUBLIC OF

IAMAT doctors available; water, milk products, and food safe

Required

None

Risks

None, recommend updating *Diphtheria, Polio* and *Tetanus* vaccines

GHANA

IAMAT doctor available; water, milk products, and cold food unsafe

Required

Yellow fever vaccine (over age one) if in infected country previous 14 days

Risks

Yellow fever, recommend vaccine

Cholera, recommend vaccine

Infectious hepatitis, recommend 2 cc gamma globulin

Typhoid, recommend vaccine

Diphtheria, Polio, Tetanus, recommend updating vaccines

Malaria, all areas, year-round, recommend chloroquine prophylaxis

GIBRALTAR

No IAMAT doctor; water probably safe but not recommended; milk products and food safe

Required

None

Risks

None, recommend updating *Diphtheria, Tetanus, Polio* vaccines

GREECE

IAMAT doctors available; water probably safe but not recommended; milk products and food safe

Required

Yellow fever vaccine (over 6 mos. old) if in infected area previous 14 days

Risks

Typhoid, recommend vaccine for those outside usual tourist areas

Diphtheria, Polio, Tetanus, recommend updating vaccines

GREENLAND

No IAMAT doctor available; water, milk products, and food safe

Required

None

Risks

None, recommend updating *Diphtheria, Polio, Tetanus* vaccines

GRENADA

No IAMAT doctor; water probably safe but not recommended; milk products and food safe

Required

None

Risks

None, recommend updating *Diphtheria, Polio, Tetanus* vaccines

GUADELOUPE

IAMAT doctor available; water probably safe but not recommended; milk products and food safe

Required

Yellow fever vaccine (over age one) if from infected country previous 14 days

Risks

Recommend updating *Diphtheria, Polio,* and *Tetanus* vaccines

Dengue, recommend anti-mosquito measures dusk to dawn

GUAM

No IAMAT doctor available; water, milk products, and food safe

Required

None

Risks

Dengue, recommend anti-mosquito measures dusk to dawn

Diphtheria, Polio, Tetanus, recommend updating vaccines

GUATEMALA

IAMAT doctor available; water, milk products, and cold food unsafe

Required

Yellow fever vaccine (over age one) if from infected country previous 14 days

Risks

Infectious hepatitis, recommend 2 cc gamma globulin

Typhus, recommend vaccine, good personal hygiene

Typhoid, recommend vaccine

Diphtheria, Polio, Tetanus, recommend updating vaccines

Malaria, all areas (except Guatemala City) under 3300 ft. (1500m) June–Nov., recommend chloroquine prophylaxis

GUIANA, FRENCH

IAMAT doctor available; water possibly safe but not recommended; milk products unsafe; food safe

Required

Yellow fever vaccine for all travelers over age one except those arriving from noninfected areas and staying less than two weeks.

Risks

Infectious hepatitis, recommend 2 cc gamma globulin

Rabies, recommend pre-exposure vaccine for those who may be exposed to mammals, avoid mammals

Typhoid, recommend vaccine

Diphtheria, Polio, Tetanus, recommend updating vaccine

Malaria, all areas, year-round, recommend chloroquine and Fansidar prophylaxis

GUINEA

No IAMAT doctor available; water, milk products, and cold food unsafe

Required

Yellow fever vaccine for all travelers over age one

Risks

Infectious hepatitis, recommend 2 cc gamma globulin

Rabies, recommend pre-exposure vaccine, avoid mammals

Typhoid, recommend vaccine

Diphtheria, Polio, Tetanus, recommend updating vaccines

Malaria, all areas, year-round, recommend chloroquine and Fansidar prophylaxis

GUINEA-BISSAU

No IAMAT doctor available; water, milk products, and cold food unsafe

Required

Yellow fever vaccine for those over age one if from infected countries previous 14 days from equatorial Africa, South America, or Central America

Risks

Infectious hepatitis, recommend 2 cc gamma globulin

Rabies, recommend pre-exposure vaccine, avoid mammals

Typhoid, recommend vaccine

Diphtheria, Polio, Tetanus, recommend updating vaccines

Malaria, all areas, year-round, recommend chloroquine prophylaxis

GUYANA

IAMAT doctor available; water probably safe but not recommended; milk products unsafe; food safe

Required

Yellow fever vaccine if from infected country previous 14 days or if from equatorial Africa, South America, or Central America

Risks

Yellow Fever, vaccine recommended

Infectious hepatitis, recommend 2 cc gamma globulin

Typhoid, recommend vaccine

Diphtheria, Polio, Tetanus, recommend updating vaccine

Malaria, in rural areas (except coastal from Georgetown to New Amsterdam, Essequibo river delta and islands) under 2970 ft. (900 m) year-round, recommend chloroquine and Fansidar prophylaxis

HAITI

IAMAT doctor available; water, milk products, and cold food unsafe

Required

Yellow fever vaccine if from infected area previous 14 days

Risks

Infectious hepatitis, recommend 5 cc gamma globulin

Typhoid, recommend vaccine

Diphtheria, Polio, Tetanus, recommend updating vaccine

Dengue, recommend anti-mosquito measures dusk to dawn

Malaria, all areas under 900 ft. (300 m), recommend chloroquine prophylaxis

HONDURAS

IAMAT doctor available; water, milk products, and cold food unsafe

Required

Yellow fever vaccine if from infected area previous 14 days

Risks

Infectious hepatitis, recommend 2 cc gamma globulin

Typhoid, recommend vaccine

Diphtheria, Polio, Tetanus, recommend updating vaccines

Malaria, all rural areas under 330 ft. (1000 m) year-round (except Octepeque Dept.), recommend chloroquine prophylaxis

HONG KONG

IAMAT doctor available; water, milk products, and cold food unsafe

Required

None

Risks

Diphteria, Polio, Tetanus, recommend updating vaccines

HUNGARY

IAMAT doctor available; water probably safe but not recommended; milk products and food safe

Required

None

Risks

Diphtheria, Polio, Tetanus, recommend updating vaccines

ICELAND

IAMAT doctor available; water, milk products, and food safe

Required

None

Risks

Diphtheria, Polio, Tetanus, recommend updating vaccines

INDIA

IAMAT doctor available; water, milk products, and cold food unsafe.

Required

Yellow fever vaccine if from infected area last 6 days or from countries in equatorial Africa, Central and South America; request *cholera vaccination* certificate if going to country demanding certificate

Risks

Cholera, recommend vaccine

Infectious hepatitis, recommend 2 cc gamma globulin

Plague, recommend vaccine or daily sulfonamide if rodent exposure likely

Rabies, recommend pre-exposure vaccine, avoid mammals

Typhus, recommend vaccine and good personal hygiene

Typhoid, recommend vaccine

Diphtheria, Polio, Tetanus, recommend updating vaccines

Dengue, apply anti-mosquito measures dusk to dawn

Malaria, all areas, year-round, recommend chloroquine and Fansidar prophylaxis

INDONESIA

IAMAT doctors available; water, milk products, and cold food unsafe

Required

Yellow fever vaccine if from infected area previous 14 days, or from equatorial Africa, Central or South America

Risks

Cholera, recommend vaccine

Infectious hepatitis, recommend 2 cc gamma globulin

Rabies, recommend pre-exposure vaccine, avoid mammals

Typhoid, recommend vaccine

Diphtheria, Polio, Tetanus, recommend updating vaccines

Dengue, apply anti-mosquito measures dusk to dawn

Malaria, all areas under 3960 ft. (1200 m) year-round, recommend chloroquine and Fansidar prophylaxis

IRAN

No IAMAT doctor available; water, milk products, and cold food unsafe.

Required

Yellow fever vaccine if from infected area previous 14 days or (over age one), if from equatorial Africa, Central or South America

Risks

Infectious hepatitis, recommend 2 cc gamma globulin

Plague, recommend vaccine if rodent exposure likely

Typhus, recommend vaccine and good personal hygiene

Typhoid, recommend vaccine

Diphtheria, Polio, Tetanus, recommend updating vaccine

Malaria, in rural areas under 4950 ft. (1500 m), July-Nov., recommend chloroquine prophylaxis

Cholera, recommend vaccine

IRAQ

IAMAT doctors available; water, milk products, and cold food unsafe

Required

Yellow fever vaccine if from infected country previous 14 days

Risks

Infectious hepatitis, recommend 2 cc gamma globulin

Plague, recommend vaccine or daily sulfonamide if rodent exposure likely

Typhus, recommend vaccine and good personal hygiene

Typhoid, recommend vaccine

Diphtheria, Polio, Tetanus, recommend updating vaccines

Malaria, May-Nov. all areas under 4950 ft. (1500 m), recommend chloroquine prophylaxis

IRELAND, NORTHERN

Same as Republic of Ireland (below)

IRELAND, REPUBLIC OF

IAMAT doctors available; water, milk products, and food safe

Required

None

Risks

Diphtheria, Polio, Tetanus, recommend updating vaccines

ISRAEL

IAMAT doctors available; water probably safe but not recommended; milk products and food safe

Required

None

Risks

Diphtheria, Polio, Tetanus, recommend updating vaccines

ITALY

IAMAT doctors available; water probably safe but not recommended; milk products and food safe

Required

None

Risks

Diphtheria, Polio, Tetanus, recommend updating vaccines

IVORY COAST

IAMAT doctor available; water, milk products, and cold food unsafe

Required

Yellow fever vaccine for all travelers over age one

Risks

Infectious hepatitis, recommend 2 cc gamma globulin

Typhoid, recommend vaccine

Diphteria, Polio, Tetanus, recommend updating vaccines

Malaria, all areas, year-round, recommend chloroquine prophylaxis

JAMAICA

IAMAT doctor available; water, probably safe but not recommended; milk products and food safe

Required

Yellow fever vaccine (over age one) if from infected country previous 14 days

Risks

Dengue, recommend anti-mosquito measures dusk to dawn

Diphtheria, Polio, Tetanus, recommend updating vaccines

JAPAN

IAMAT doctors available; water, milk products, and food safe

Required

None

Risks

Diphtheria, Polio, Tetanus, recommend updating vaccine

JORDAN

IAMAT doctors available; water, milk products, and cold food unsafe

Required

None

Risks

Infectious hepatitis, recommend 2 cc gamma globulin

Typhoid, recommend vaccine

Diphtheria, Polio, Tetanus, recommend updating vaccines

Malaria, April–Nov. in rural Jordan River Valley and Kerak lowlands, recommend chloroquine prophylaxis

Cholera, recommend vaccine

KAMPUCHEA PEOPLE'S REPUBLIC (CAMBODIA)

No IAMAT doctor; water, milk products, and cold food unsafe

Required

Yellow fever vaccine if from infected country previous 14 days

Risks

Infectious hepatitis, recommend 2 cc gamma globulin

Plague, recommend vaccine if wild rodent exposure likely

Typhoid, recommend vaccine

Diphtheria, Polio, Tetanus, recommend updating vaccine

Dengue, recommend anti-mosquito measures dusk to dawn

Malaria, recommend chloroquine and Fansidar prophylaxis

KENYA

IAMAT doctor available; water unsafe; milk products probably safe; cold food unsafe

Required

Yellow fever vaccine if from infected country previous 14 days, or those over age one from equatorial Africa, Central or South America

Risks

Yellow fever, recommend vaccine

Infectious hepatitis, recommend 2 cc gamma globulin

Typhoid, recommend vaccine

Diphtheria, Polio, Tetanus, recommend updating vaccines

KIRIBATI (GILBERT ISLANDS)

No IAMAT doctors available; water, milk products, and cold food unsafe

Required

Yellow fever vaccine (those over age one) if from infected country last 14 days

Risks

Infectious hepatitis, recommend 2 cc gamma globulin

Typhoid, recommend vaccine

Diphtheria, Polio, Tetanus, recommend updating vaccines

Dengue, recommend anti-mosquito measures dusk to dawn

KOREA, DEM. PEOPLE'S REPUBLIC OF (NORTH KOREA)

No IAMAT doctor available; water, milk products, and cold food unsafe

Required

None

Risks

Infectious hepatitis, recommend 2 cc gamma globulin

Typhoid, recommend vaccine

Diphtheria, Polio, Tetanus, recommend updating vaccines

KOREA, REPUBLIC OF (SOUTH KOREA)

IAMAT doctor available; water, milk products, and cold food unsafe

Required

Yellow fever vaccine (over age one) if from infected country previous 14 days

Risks

Infectious Hepatitis, recommend 2 cc gamma globulin

Typhoid, recommend vaccine

Diphtheria, Polio, Tetanus, recommend updating vaccines

KUWAIT

IAMAT doctor available; water probably safe but not recommended; milk products and food safe

Required

None

Risks

Diphtheria, Polio, Tetanus, recommend updating vaccines

LAO, PEOPLE'S DEMOCRATIC REPUBLIC (LAOS)

No IAMAT doctor available; water, milk products, and cold food unsafe

Required

Yellow fever vaccine if from infected country previous 14 days

Risks

Infectious hepatitis, recommend 2 cc gamma globulin

Plague, recommend vaccine or daily sulfonamide prophylaxis if wild rodent exposures likely

Typhoid, recommend vaccine

Diphtheria, Polio, Tetanus, recommend updating vaccines

Dengue, recommend anti-mosquito measures dusk to dawn

Malaria, all areas (except Vientiane) year-round, recommend chloroquine and Fansidar prophylaxis

LEBANON

IAMAT doctor available; water, probably safe but not recommended; milk products and cold food safe

Required

Yellow fever vaccine if from infected country previous 14 days

Risks

Diphtheria, Polio, Tetanus, recommend updating vaccines

LESOTHO

IAMAT doctor available; water, milk products, and food safe

Required

Cholera vaccine and *Yellow fever vaccine* if from infected countries previous 14 days

Risks

Infectious hepatitis, recommend 2 cc gamma globulin

Plague, recommend vaccine of sulfonamide prophylaxis if wild rodent exposure likely

Typhoid, recommend vaccine

Diphtheria, Polio, Tetanus, recommend updating vaccines

LIBERIA

IAMAT doctor available; water, milk products, and cold food unsafe.

Required

Yellow fever vaccine (over age one) if from infected country previous 14 days or if from equatorial Africa, South or Central America

Risks

Cholera, Recommend vaccine

Yellow fever, recommend vaccine

Infectious hepatitis, recommend 2 cc gamma globulin

Typhoid, recommend vaccine

Diphtheria, Polio, Tetanus, recommend updating vaccines

Malaria, all areas, year-round, recommend chloroquine prophylaxis

LIBYAN ARAB JAMAHIRIYA
(Formerly Libyan Arab Republic)

IAMAT doctor available; water, milk products, and cold food unsafe

Required

Cholera vaccine if from infected country previous 14 days; *Yellow fever vaccine* (over age one) if from infected country previous 14 days.

Risks

Infectious hepatitis, recommend 2 cc gamma globulin

Typhoid, recommend vaccine

Diphtheria, Polio, Tetanus, recommend updating vaccines

Malaria, in rural areas of southwest Feb.–Aug., recommend chloroquine prophylaxis

LIECHTENSTEIN

IAMAT doctor available; water, milk products, and food safe

Required

None

Risks

Diphtheria, Polio, Tetanus, recommend updating vaccines

LUXEMBOURG

IAMAT doctor available; water, milk products, and food safe

Required

None

Risks

Diphtheria, Polio, Tetanus, recommend updating vaccines

MACAO

IAMAT doctor available; water, milk products, and cold food unsafe

Required

None

Risks

Diphtheria, Polio, Tetanus, recommend updating vaccines

MADAGASCAR

No IAMAT doctor available; water, milk products, and cold food unsafe.

Required

Cholera (over age 6 months) and *Yellow fever vaccines* (over age one) if from infected country previous 14 days

Risks

Infectious hepatitis, recommend 2 cc gamma globulin

Plague, recommend vaccine or sulfa prophylaxis if wild rodent exposure likely

Typhoid, recommend vaccine

Diphtheria, Polio, Tetanus, recommend updating vaccines

Malaria, most areas under 3630 ft. (1100 m) Sept.–March, recommend chloroquine and Fansidar prophylaxis

MADEIRA ISLANDS

IAMAT doctor available; water probably safe but not recommended; milk products and cold food safe

Required

Yellow fever vaccine (those over age one) from infected country previous 14 days

Risks

Diphtheria, Polio, Tetanus, recommend updating vaccines

MALAWI

IAMAT doctor available; water, milk products, and cold food unsafe

Required

Yellow fever vaccine (those over age one) if from infected country previous 14 days

Risks

Yellow fever, recommend vaccine

Typhoid, recommend vaccine

Diphtheria, Polio, Tetanus, recommend updating vaccines

Malaria, all areas, year-round, recommend chloroquine prophylaxis

MALAYSIA

IAMAT doctor available; water, milk products, and cold food unsafe

Required

Yellow fever vaccine (those over age one) if from infected country previous 14 days or from equatorial Africa, South and Central America

Risks

Cholera, recommend immunization

Infectious hepatitis, recommend 2 cc gamma globulin

Typhoid, recommend vaccine

Diphtheria, Polio, Tetanus, recommend updating vaccines

Dengue, recommend anti-mosquito measures dusk to dawn

Malaria, in all areas under 5610 ft. (1700 m) except coastal Malaya peninsula and Sarawak) year-round, recommend chloroquine and Fansidar prophylaxis

MALDIVES

No IAMAT doctor available; water, milk products, and cold food unsafe

Required

Cholera vaccine for all travelers, *Yellow fever vaccine* if from infected country previous 14 days

Risks

Infectious hepatitis, recommend 2 cc gamma globulin

Typhoid, recommend vaccine

Diphtheria, Polio, Tetanus, recommend updating vaccine

Malaria, all areas except Male Island, year-round, recommend chloroquine prophylaxis

MALI

No IAMAT doctor available; water, milk products, and cold food unsafe.

Required

Cholera vaccine if from infected country previous 14 days; *Yellow fever vaccine* unless arrive from noninfected area and staying less than two weeks

Risks

Yellow fever, recommend vaccine

Infectious hepatitis, recommend 2 cc gamma globulin

Typhoid, recommend vaccine

Diphtheria, Polio, Tetanus, recommend updating vaccines

Malaria, all areas, year-round, recommend chloroquine prophylaxis

MALTA

IAMAT doctor available; water probably safe but not recommended; milk products and food safe

Required

Cholera vaccine if from infected country previous 14 days, *Yellow fever vaccine* (those over age 6 months) if from infected country previous 14 days

Risks

Diphtheria, Polio, Tetanus, recommend updating vaccines

MARTINIQUE

IAMAT doctor available; water probably safe but not recommended; milk products and food safe

Required

Yellow fever vaccine (those over age one) if from infected country previous 14 days

Risks

Diphtheria, Polio, Tetanus, recommend updating vaccines

Dengue, recommend anti-mosquito measures dusk to dawn

MAURITANIA

No IAMAT doctor available; water, milk products, and cold food unsafe

Required

Yellow fever vaccine for all travelers over age one, only exception is if from noninfected area and staying less than two weeks

Risks

Infectious hepatitis, recommend 2 cc gamma globulin

Rabies, recommend pre-exposure rabies vaccine, avoid contact with mammals

Typhoid, recommend vaccine

Diphtheria, Polio, Tetanus, recommend updating vaccines

Malaria, in all areas, recommend chloroquine prophylaxis

MAURITIUS

No IAMAT doctor available; water, milk products, and cold food unsafe.

Required

Yellow fever vaccine (those over age one) if from infected country previous 14 days or from equatorial Africa, Central or South America

Risks

Diphtheria, Polio, Tetanus, recommend updating vaccines

MEXICO

IAMAT doctors available; water unsafe, milk products, and cold food unsafe.

Required

Yellow fever vaccine (those over 6 months old) if in infected country during preceding 14 days

Risks

Infectious hepatitis, recommend 2 cc gamma globulin

Typhoid, recommend vaccine if outside tourist areas or working there

Polio, Tetanus, Diphtheria, update vaccines

Dengue, recommend mosquito repellent, screen and/or mosquito nets

MONACO

IAMAT doctor available; water probably safe but not recommended; milk products and food safe

Required

None

Risks

Diphtheria, Polio, Tetanus, recommend updating vaccines

MONGOLIA

No IAMAT doctor available; water, milk products, and cold food unsafe

Required

None

Risks

Diphtheria, Polio, Tetanus, recommend updating vaccines

MONTSERRAT

No IAMAT doctor available; water probably safe but not recommended; milk products and food safe

Required

Yellow fever vaccine (those over age one) if from infected country previous 14 days

Risks

Diphtheria, Polio, Tetanus, recommend updating vaccines

MOROCCO

IAMAT doctor available; water, milk products, and cold food unsafe

Required

None

Risks

Infectious hepatitis, recommend 2 cc gamma globulin

Rabies, recommend pre-exposure vaccine, avoid mammals

Typhoid, recommend vaccine

Diphtheria, Polio, Tetanus, recommend updating vaccines

Malaria, rural areas, May–Oct., recommend chloroquine prophylaxis

MOZAMBIQUE

No IAMAT doctor available; water, milk products, and cold food unsafe

Required

Cholera vaccine; Yellow fever vaccine (those over age one) if from infected area previous 14 days

Risks

Infectious hepatitis, recommend 2 cc gamma globulin

Plague, recommend vaccine or daily sulfa if wild rodent exposure likely

Rabies, recommend pre-exposure vaccine, avoid mammals

Typhoid, recommend vaccine

Diphtheria, Polio, Tetanus, recommend updating vaccines

Malaria, all areas, year-round, recommend chloroquine prophylaxis

NAMIBIA

No IAMAT doctor available; water probably safe but not recommended; milk products and food safe

Required

Yellow fever vaccine if from infected area previous 14 days, or from Africa, Central or South America; some exclusions, e.g., airline passengers not from infected areas who do not leave airport or adjacent town

Risks

Infectious hepatitis, recommend 2 cc gamma globulin

Plague, recommend vaccine or daily sulfa if wild rodent exposure likely

Typhoid, recommend vaccine

Diphtheria, Polio, Tetanus, recommend updating vaccines

Malaria, recommend chloroquine prophylaxis

NAURU ISLAND

No IAMAT doctor available; water, milk products, and cold food unsafe

Required

Yellow fever vaccine (those over age one) if from infected country previous 14 days

Risks

Diphtheria, Polio, Tetanus, recommend updating vaccines

Dengue, recommend anti-mosquito measures dusk to dawn

NEPAL

IAMAT doctor available; water, milk products, and cold food unsafe.

Required

Yellow fever vaccine if from infected country previous 14 days.

Risks

Cholera, recommend vaccine

Infectious hepatitis, recommend 2 cc gamma globulin

Plague, recommend vaccine or daily sulfonamide if wild rodent exposure likely

Rabies, recommend pre-exposure vaccine, avoid mammals

Typhus, recommend vaccine

Typhoid, recommend vaccine

Diphtheria, Tetanus, Polio, recommend updating vaccines

Malaria, all areas under 3900 ft. (1200 m) year-round, recommend chloroquine prophylaxis.

NETHERLANDS

IAMAT doctor available; water, milk products, and food safe.

Required

None

Risks

Diphtheria, Polio, Tetanus, recommend updating vaccines

NETHERLANDS ANTILLES

IAMAT doctor available; water probably safe but not recommended; milk products and food safe

Required

Yellow fever vaccine, (those over 6 months) if from infected country previous 14 days

Risks

Diphtheria, Polio, Tetanus, recommend updating vaccines

NEW CALEDONIA AND DEPENDENCIES

No IAMAT doctor available; water probably safe but not recommended; milk products and food safe

Required

Yellow fever vaccine (those over age 6 months) if from infected country previous 14 days or from equatorial Africa, Central or South America

Risks

Infectious hepatitis, recommend 2 cc gamma globulin

Typhoid, recommend vaccine

Diphtheria, Polio, Tetanus, recommend updating vaccines

Dengue, recommend anti-mosquito measures dusk to dawn

NEW ZEALAND

IAMAT doctor available; water, milk products, and food safe.

Required

None

Risks

Diphtheria, Polio, Tetanus, recommend updating vaccines

NICARAGUA

No IAMAT doctor available; water, milk products, and cold food unsafe

Required

None

Risks

Infectious hepatitis, recommend 2 cc gamma globulin

Typhoid, recommend vaccine

Diphtheria, Polio, Tetanus, recommend updating vaccines

Malaria, most areas under 3300 ft. (100 m) May–Dec., recommend chloroquine prophylaxis

NIGER

IAMAT doctor available; water, milk products, and cold food unsafe

Required

Yellow fever vaccine (those over age one) and *cholera vaccine* if from infected country previous 14 days

Risks

Infectious hepatitis, recommend 2 cc gamma globulin

Typhus, recommend vaccine and good personal hygiene

Typhoid, recommend vaccine

Diphtheria, Polio, Tetanus, recommend updating vaccines

Malaria, all areas, year-round, recommend chloroquine prophylaxis

NIGERIA

IAMAT doctor available; water, milk products, and cold food unsafe.

Required

Yellow fever vaccine (those over age one), *cholera vaccine* if going to country requiring it

Risks

Cholera, recommend vaccine

Infectious hepatitis, recommend 2 cc gamma globulin

Rabies, recommend pre-exposure vaccine, avoid mammals

Typhus, recommend vaccine

Typhoid, recommend vaccine

Diphtheria, Polio, Tetanus, recommend updating vaccines

Malaria, all areas, year-round, recommend chloroquine prophylaxis

NIUE ISLANDS

No IAMAT doctor available; water probably safe but not recommended; milk products and food safe

Required

Yellow fever vaccine (those over age one) if from infected country previous 14 days

Risks

Diphtheria, Polio, Tetanus, recommend updating vaccines

Dengue, recommend anti-mosquito measures dusk to dawn

NORWAY

IAMAT doctor available; water, milk products, and food safe

Required

None

Risks

Diphtheria, Polio, Tetanus, recommend updating vaccines

OMAN

IAMAT doctor available; water, milk products, and cold food unsafe.

Required

None

Risks

Infectious hepatitis, recommended 2 cc gamma globulin

Typhoid, recommend vaccine

Diphtheria, Polio, Tetanus, recommend updating vaccines

Malaria, all areas, year-round, recommend chloroquine prophylaxis

PAKISTAN

IAMAT doctor available; water, milk products, and cold food unsafe

Required

Cholera vaccine; *Yellow fever vaccine* if from infected country previous 14 days or from equatorial Africa, Central or South America

Risks

Infectious hepatitis, recommend 2 cc gamma globulin

Rabies, recommend pre-exposure vaccine, avoid mammals

Typhus, recommend vaccine and good personal hygiene

Typhoid, recommend vaccine

Diphtheria, Polio, Tetanus, recommend updating vaccines

Malaria, all areas, year-round, recommend chloroquine prophylaxis

PANAMA

IAMAT doctor available; water, milk products, and cold food unsafe.

Required

None

Risks

Yellow Fever, recommend vaccine

Infectious hepatitis, recommend 2 cc gamma globulin

Typhoid, recommend vaccine

Diphtheria, Polio, Tetanus, recommend updating vaccines

Malaria, in certain rural areas under 2640 ft (800 m), year-round, chloroquine and Fansidar prophylaxis recommended

PAPUA NEW GUINEA

IAMAT doctor available; water and cold food unsafe; milk products safe

Required

Yellow fever vaccine if from infected country previous 14 days.

Risks

Infectious hepatitis, recommend 2 cc gamma globulin

Typhoid, recommend vaccine

Diphtheria, Polio, Tetanus, recommend updating vaccines

Malaria, all areas, year-round, recommend chloroquine and Fansidar prophylaxis

PARAGUAY

IAMAT doctor available; water, milk products, and cold food unsafe

Required

Yellow fever vaccine (those over 6 mos. of age) if from infected country previous 14 days; *Cholera vaccine* if from infected area

Risks

Infectious hepatitis, recommend 2 cc gamma globulin

Typhoid, recommend vaccine

Diphtheria, Polio, Tetanus, recommend updating vaccines

Malaria, in rural areas bordering Brazil, Oct.–May, recommend chloroquine prophylaxis

PERU

IAMAT doctor available; water, milk products, and cold food unsafe

Required

Yellow fever vaccine (those over 6 mos. of age) if from infected country previous 14 days

Risks

Yellow Fever, recommend vaccine

Infectious hepatitis, recommend 2 cc gamma globulin

Plague, recommend vaccine or daily sulfonamide if exposure to wild rodents likely

Typhus, recommend vaccine

Typhoid, recommend vaccine

Diphtheria, Polio, Tetanus, recommend updating vaccines

Malaria, in all areas (except Lima) under 4950 ft. (1500 m), recommend chloroquine and Fansidar prophylaxis

Violence, don't travel alone in rural areas

PHILIPPINES

IAMAT doctor available; water, milk products, and cold food unsafe.

Required

Yellow fever vaccine (those over age one) if from infected area previous 6 days.

Risks

Cholera, recommend vaccine

Infectious hepatitis, recommend 2 cc gamma globulin

Rabies, recommend pre-exposure vaccine, avoid mammals

Typhoid, recommend vaccine

Diphtheria, Polio, Tetanus recommend updating vaccines

Dengue, anti-mosquito measures dusk to dawn

Malaria, in most rural areas under 1980 ft. (600 m), year-round, recommend chloroquine and Fansidar prophylaxis

PITCAIRN ISLAND

No IAMAT doctor available; water probably safe but not recommended; milk products safety unknown; food safe

Required

Cholera vaccine; *Yellow fever vaccine* (those over age one) if from infected country previous 14 days

Risks

Diphtheria, Polio, Tetanus, recommend updating vaccines

Dengue, anti-mosquito measures dusk to dawn

POLAND

IAMAT doctor available; water probably safe but not recommended; milk products and food safe

Required

None

Risks

Diphtheria, Polio, Tetanus, recommend updating vaccines

POLYNESIA, FRENCH
(Tahiti, Society islands; Marquesas Island; Tuamotu archipelago, Gambier islands, Austral islands)

IAMAT doctor available in Tahiti; water probably safe but not recommended; milk products and food safe

Required

Yellow fever vaccine (those over age one) if from infected country previous 14 days

Risks

Diphtheria, Polio, Tetanus, recommended updating vaccines

Dengue, recommend anti-mosquito measures dusk to dawn

PORTUGAL

IAMAT doctor available; water probably safe but not recommended; milk products and food safe

Required

Yellow fever vaccine if from infected country previous 14 days or from equatorial Africa, Central or South America, and destined for Azores and Maderia

Risks

Diphtheria, Polio, Tetanus, recommend updating vaccines

PUERTO RICO

IAMAT doctor available; water, milk products, and food safe

Required

None

Risks

Diphtheria, Polio, Tetanus, recommend updating vaccines

Dengue, recommend anti-mosquito measures dusk to dawn

QATAR

No IAMAT doctor available; water, milk products, and cold food unsafe

Required

Yellow fever vaccine (those over age one) if from infected country previous 14 days

Risks

Infectious Hepatitis, recommend 2 cc gamma globulin

Typhoid, recommend vaccine

Diphtheria, Polio, Tetanus, recommend updating vaccines

RÉUNION

No IAMAT doctor available; water, milk products, and cold food unsafe

Required

Yellow fever vaccine (those over age one) if from infected country previous 14 days.

Risks

Diphtheria, Polio, Tetanus, recommend updating vaccines

ROMANIA

No IAMAT doctor available; water probably safe but not recommended; milk products and food safe

Required

None

Risks

Diphtheria, Polio, Tetanus, recommend updating vaccines

RWANDA

IAMAT doctor available; water, milk products, and cold food safe

Required

Yellow fever vaccine if from infected country previous 14 days

Risks

Cholera, recommend vaccine

Yellow fever, recommend vaccine

Typhus, recommend vaccine

Infectious hepatitis, recommend 2 cc gamma globulin

Typhoid, recommend vaccine

Diphtheria, Polio, Tetanus, recommend updating vaccines

Malaria, in all areas, year-round, recommend chloroquine prophylaxis

SAINT HELENA

No IAMAT doctor available; water probably safe but not recommended; milk products and food safe

Required

None

Risks

Diphtheria, Polio, Tetanus, recommend updating vaccine

ST. KITTS-NEVIS, ANGUILLA

No IAMAT doctor available; water probably safe but not recommended; milk products and food safe

Required

Yellow fever vaccine (those over age one) if from infected country previous 14 days

Risks

Diphtheria, Polio, Tetanus, recommend updating vaccines

SAINT LUCIA

IAMAT doctor available; water probably safe but not recommended; milk products and food safe

Required

Yellow fever vaccine (those over age one) if from infected country previous 14 days or from equatorial Africa, Central or South America.

Risks

Diphtheria, Polio, Tetanus, recommend updating vaccines

ST. PIERRE AND MIQUELON

No IAMAT doctor available; water probably safe but not recommended; milk products and food safe

Required

None

Risks

Diphtheria, Polio, Tetanus, recommend updating vaccines

ST. VINCENT

No IAMAT doctor available; water probably safe but not recommended; milk products and food safe

Required

Yellow fever vaccine (those over age one) if from infected country previous 14 days or from equatorial Africa, Central or South America

Risks

Diphtheria, Polio, Tetanus, recommend updating vaccines

SAMOA, AMERICAN

No IAMAT doctor available; water probably safe but not recommended; milk products and food safe

Required

Yellow fever vaccine (those over age one) if from infected country previous 14 days

Risks

Diphtheria, Polio, Tetanus, recommend updating vaccines

Dengue, recommend anti-mosquito measures dusk to dawn

SAMOA, WESTERN

No IAMAT doctor available; water probably safe but not recommended; milk products and food safe

Required

Yellow fever vaccine (those over age one) if from infected country previous 14 days

Risks

Diphtheria, Polio, Tetanus, recommend updating vaccines

Dengue, recommend anti-mosquito measures dusk to dawn

SAO TOME AND PRINCIPE

No IAMAT doctor available; water, milk products, and cold food unsafe

Required

Yellow fever vaccine (those over age one) for all travelers except from noninfected areas staying less than 2 weeks

Risks

Yellow fever, recommend vaccine

Infectious hepatitis, recommend 2 cc gamma globulin

Typhoid, recommend updating vaccine

Diphtheria, Polio, Tetanus, recommend updating vaccines

Malaria, all areas, year-round, recommend chloroquine prophylaxis

SAUDI ARABIA

IAMAT doctor available; water, milk products, and cold food unsafe

Required

Yellow fever vaccine for all travelers if from infected country previous 14 days

Risks

Infectious hepatitis, recommend 2 cc gamma globulin

Typhoid, recommend vaccine

Diphtheria, Polio, Tetanus, recommend updating vaccines

Malaria, in most areas year-round, recommend chloroquine prophylaxis (except in Alkosa, Arar, Jauf, Quraiya, Riyadh, Tebuk, Taif)

SCOTLAND

IAMAT doctor available; see United Kingdom (below)

SENEGAL

IAMAT doctor available; water, milk products, and cold food unsafe

Required

Yellow fever vaccine (those over age one)

Risks

Infectious hepatitis, recommend 2 cc gamma globulin

Typhoid, recommend vaccine

Diphtheria, Polio, Tetanus, recommend updating vaccine

Malaria, all areas, year-round, recommend chloroquine prophylaxis

SEYCHELLES

No IAMAT doctor available; water probably safe but not recommended; milk products and food safe

Required

None

Risks

Diphtheria, Polio, Tetanus, recommend updating vaccines

SIERRA LEONE

IAMAT doctor available; water, milk products, and cold food unsafe

Required

Yellow fever vaccine may be required when leaving country

Risks

Yellow fever, recommend vaccine

Infectious hepatitis, recommend 2 cc gamma globulin

Rabies, recommend pre-exposure vaccine, avoid mammals

Typhoid, recommend vaccine

Diphtheria, Polio, Tetanus, recommend updating vaccines

Malaria, all areas, year-round, recommend chloroquine prophylaxis

SINGAPORE

IAMAT doctor available; water probably safe but not recommended; milk products and food safe

Required

Yellow fever vaccine (those over age one), if from infected country previous 14 days, or if from equatorial Africa, Central or South America

Risks

Diphtheria, Polio, Tetanus, recommend updating vaccine

Dengue, recommend anti-mosquito measures dusk to dawn

Malaria, in rural areas on northern part of main island, Chiangi Village and offshore islands, year-round, recommend chloroquine prophylaxis

SOLOMON ISLANDS

No IAMAT doctors available; water probably safe but not recommended; milk products and food safe

Required

Yellow fever vaccine if from infected country previous 14 days

Risks

Diphtheria, Polio, Tetanus, recommend updating vaccines

Dengue, recommend anti-mosquito measures dusk to dawn

Malaria, in most areas under 1320 ft. (400 m) year-round, recommend chloroquine and Fansidar prophylaxis

SOMALIA

No IAMAT doctor available; water, milk products, and cold food unsafe

Required

Cholera vaccine and *Yellow fever vaccine* if from infected country previous 14 days.

Risks

Yellow fever, recommend vaccine

Infectious hepatitis, recommend 2 cc gamma globulin

Typhoid, recommend vaccine

Diphtheria, *Polio*, *Tetanus*, recommend updating vaccines

Dengue, recommend anti-mosquito measures dusk to dawn

Malaria, in all areas, year-round, recommend chloroquine prophylaxis (low risk in Magadisku)

SOUTH AFRICA, REPUBLIC OF

IAMAT doctor available; water, milk products, and food safe

Required

Yellow fever vaccine if from infected country previous 14 days or from equatorial Africa, Central or South America (excluding scheduled commercial airline passengers from and to noninfected areas who remain in the airport or adjacent town during transit)

Risks

Infectious hepatitis, recommend vaccine if traveling outside usual tourist areas

Plague, recommend vaccine or daily sulfonamide prophylaxis if wild rodent exposure likely

Typhus, recommend vaccine and good personal hygiene if in interior

Typhoid, recommend vaccine

Diphtheria, *Polio*, *Tetanus*, recommend updating vaccines

Malaria, in areas under 3960 ft. (1200 m) bordering other countries, i.e., Botswana, Mozambique, Zimbabwe year-round, recommend chloroquine prophylaxis

SPAIN

IAMAT doctor available; water probably safe but not recommended; milk products and food safe

Required

None

Risks

Diphtheria, Polio, Tetanus, recommend updating vaccine

SRI LANKA

IAMAT doctor available; water, milk products, and cold food unsafe

Required

Yellow fever vaccine (those over age one) if from infected country or equatorial Africa, Central or South America previous 14 days

Risks

Cholera, recommend vaccine

Infectious hepatitis, recommend 2 cc gamma globulin

Rabies, recommend pre-exposure vaccine, avoid mammals

Typhoid, recommend vaccine

Diphtheria, Polio, Tetanus, recommend updating vaccines

Dengue, recommend anti-mosquito measures dusk to dawn

Malaria, most areas except Colombo under 2640 ft. (800 m), year-round, recommend chloroquine prophylaxis

SUDAN

IAMAT doctor available; water, milk products, and cold food unsafe

Required

Yellow fever vaccine (those under age one) if from infected country previous 14 days or from equatorial Africa, Central or South America; *Cholera vaccine* if from infected country previous 14 days

Risks

Yellow fever, recommend vaccine

Infectious hepatitis, recommend 2 cc gamma globulin

Plague, recommend vaccine if outside usual tourist areas

Rabies, recommend pre-exposure vaccine, avoid mammals

Typhoid, recommend vaccine

Diphtheria, Tetanus, Polio, recommend updating vaccines

Malaria, all areas, year-round, recommend chloroquine prophylaxis

SURINAM

IAMAT doctor available; water probably safe but not recommended; milk products unsafe; food safe

Required

Yellow fever vaccine if from infected country previous 14 days

Risks

Yellow fever, recommend vaccine

Infectious hepatitis, recommend 2 cc gamma globulin

Typhoid, recommend vaccine

Diphtheria, Polio, Tetanus, recommend updating vaccines

Malaria, in rural areas (except Paramaribo district and coastal areas north of 5°N) year-round, recommend chloroquine and Fansidar prophylaxis

SWAZILAND

IAMAT doctor available; water, milk products, and food safe

Required

Cholera and *Yellow fever vaccines* if from infected country previous 14 days

Risks

Infectious hepatitis, recommend 2 cc gamma globulin

Plague, recommend vaccine or daily sulfonamide if wild rodent exposure likely

Rabies, recommend pre-exposure vaccine, avoid mammals

Typhus, recommend vaccine and good personal hygiene if in interior

Typhoid, recommend vaccine

Diphtheria, Polio, Tetanus, recommend updating vaccines

Malaria, northern border areas, Dec.–March, recommend chloroquine prophylaxis

SWEDEN

IAMAT doctor available; water, milk products, and food safe

Required

None

Risks

Diphtheria, Polio, Tetanus, recommend updating vaccines

SWITZERLAND

IAMAT doctor available; water, milk products, and food safe

Required

None

Risks

Diphtheria, Tetanus, Polio, recommend updating vaccines

SYRIAN ARAB REPUBLIC (SYRIA)

IAMAT doctor available; water possibly safe but not recommended; milk products and cold food unsafe.

Required

Yellow fever vaccine if from infected country previous 14 days

Risks

Cholera, vaccine recommended

Infectious hepatitis, recommend 2 cc gamma globulin

Plague, recommend vaccine or daily sulfonamide if wild rodent exposure likely

Typhoid, recommend vaccine

Diphtheria, *Polio*, *Tetanus*, recommend updating vaccines

Dengue, recommend anti-mosquito measures dusk to dawn

Malaria, in most rural areas under 1980 ft. (600 m) May–Oct., recommend chloroquine prophylaxis

TANZANIA, UNITED REPUBLIC OF

IAMAT doctor available; water, milk products, and cold food unsafe

Required

Yellow fever vaccine (those over age one) if from infected area previous 14 days or from equatorial Africa, Central or South America

Risks

Cholera, recommend vaccine

Infectious hepatitis, recommend 2 cc gamma globulin

Yellow fever, recommend vaccine

Plague, recommend vaccine or daily sulfonamide if wild rodent exposure likely

Rabies, recommend pre-exposure vaccine, avoid mammals

Typhoid, recommend vaccine

Diphtheria, *Polio*, *Tetanus*, recommend updating vaccines

Malaria, all areas, year-round, recommend chloroquine and Fansidar prophylaxis

THAILAND

IAMAT doctor available; water, milk products, and cold food unsafe

Required

Yellow fever vaccine (those over age one) if from infected country previous 14 days or from equatorial Africa, Central or South America

Risks

Cholera, recommend vaccine

Infectious hepatitis, recommend 2 cc gamma globulin

Rabies, recommend pre-exposure vaccine, avoid mammals

Typhoid, recommend vaccine

Diphtheria, *Polio*, *Tetanus*, recommend updating vaccines

Dengue, recommend anti-mosquito measures dusk to dawn

Malaria, all rural areas, year-round, recommend chloroquine and Fansidar prophylaxis

TOGO

No IAMAT doctor available; water, milk products, and cold food unsafe

Required

Yellow fever vaccine (those over age one) if from infected country previous 14 days

Risks

Yellow fever, recommend vaccine

Infectious hepatitis, recommend 2 cc gamma globulin

Typhus, recommend vaccine if in interior, also good personal hygiene

Typhoid, recommend vaccine

Diphtheria, *Polio*, *Tetanus*, recommend updating vaccines

Malaria, all areas, year-round, recommend chloroquine prophylaxis

TONGA

IAMAT doctor available; water probably safe but not recommended; milk products and food safe

Required

Yellow fever vaccine (those over age one) if from infected country previous 14 days

Risks

Diphtheria, Polio, Tetanus, recommend updating vaccines

Dengue, recommend anti-mosquito measures dusk to dawn

TRINIDAD AND TOBAGO

IAMAT doctor available; water probably safe but not recommended; milk products and food safe

Required

Yellow fever vaccine (those over age one) if from infected country previous 14 days

Risks

Yellow fever, recommend vaccine if outside usual tourist areas

Diphtheria, Polio, Tetanus, recommend updating vaccine

TUNISIA

IAMAT doctor available; water may be safe in some cities but not recommended; milk products and cold food unsafe

Required

Yellow fever vaccine (those over age one) if from infected country previous 14 days

Risks

Infectious hepatitis, recommend 2 cc gamma globulin

Typhoid, recommend vaccine

Diphtheria, Polio, Tetanus, recommend updating vaccines

Malaria, in northern rural areas May-Nov., recommend chloroquine prophylaxis

TURKEY

IAMAT doctor available; water unsafe in Middle East but may be safe in European Turkey (Istanbul, Edirne) but not recommended; milk products and cold food unsafe in Middle East but safe in European Turkey

Required

None

Risks

Infectious hepatitis, recommend 2 cc gamma globulin

Rabies, recommend pre-exposure vaccine, avoid mammals

Typhoid, recommend vaccine

Diphtheria, Polio, Tetanus, recommend updating vaccines

Dengue, recommend anti-mosquito measures dusk to dawn

Malaria, in many areas March-Oct., recommend chloroquine prophylaxis.

TUVALU (formerly Ellice Islands)

No IAMAT doctor available; water, milk products, and cold food unsafe

Required

Yellow fever vaccine (those over age one) if from infected country previous 14 days

Risks

Diphtheria, Polio, Tetanus, recommend updating vaccines

UGANDA

IAMAT doctor available; water, milk products, and cold food unsafe

Required

Yellow fever vaccine (those over age one)

Risks

Cholera, recommend vaccine

Infectious hepatitis, recommend 2 cc gamma globulin

Rabies, recommend pre-exposure vaccine, avoid mammals

Typhoid, recommend vaccine

Diphtheria, Polio, Tetanus, recommend updating vaccines

Malaria, all areas under 5940 ft. (1800 m), year-round, recommend chloroquine prophylaxis

UNION OF SOVIET SOCIALIST REPUBLICS

No IAMAT doctor available; water unsafe; milk products safe; cold food may be safe but not recommended

Required

None

Risks

Infectious hepatitis, recommend 2 cc gamma globulin

Plague, recommend vaccine or daily sulfonamides if wild rodent exposure likely

Typhus, recommend vaccine and good hygiene

Typhoid, recommend vaccine

Diphtheria, Polio, Tetanus, recommend updating vaccine

Malaria, in a few areas near Iran and Afganistan; no risk in usual tourist areas, data incomplete; recommend chloroquine prophylaxis only if in infected area

UNITED ARAB EMIRATES (formerly Trucial States)

No IAMAT doctor available; water, milk products, and cold food unsafe

Required

Yellow fever and *cholera vaccine* if from infected country previous 14 days

Risks

Cholera, recommend vaccine

Infectious hepatitis, recommend 2 cc gamma globulin

Typhoid, recommend vaccine

Diphtheria, Polio, Tetanus, recommend updating vaccines

Malaria, all areas, year-round, recommend chloroquine prophylaxis

UNITED KINGDOM

IAMAT doctor available in Scotland and Ireland, none in England; water, milk products, and food safe

Required

None

Risks

Diphtheria, Polio, Tetanus, recommend updating vaccines

UNITED STATES OF AMERICA

No IAMAT doctor available; water, milk products, and food safe

Required

None

Risks

Diphtheria, Polio, Tetanus, recommend updating vaccines

Plague, recommend vaccine or daily sulfonamide if exposure to wild rodents likely in interiors of Arizona, California, Colorado, New Mexico or Oregon

Expensive Medical Care, recommend obtaining medical insurance coverage before travel to U.S.

URUGUAY

IAMAT doctor available; water, milk products, and food safe

Required

None

Risks

Diphtheria, Polio, Tetanus, recommend updating vaccines

VANUATU (formerly New Hebrides)

No IAMAT doctor available; water probably safe but not recommended; milk products and food safe

Required

None

Risks

Infectious hepatitis, recommend 2 cc gamma globulin

Typhoid, recommend vaccine

Diphtheria, *Polio*, *Tetanus*, recommend updating vaccines

Dengue, recommend anti-mosquito measures dusk to dawn

Malaria, in all areas (except Futuna Island) year-round, recommend chloroquine prophylaxis

VENEZUELA

IAMAT doctor available; water probably safe but not recommended; milk products and food safe

Required

None

Risks

Yellow fever, recommend vaccine

Infectious hepatitis, recommend 2 cc gamma globulin

Plague, recommend vaccine or daily sulfonamides if wild rodent exposure likely

Typhoid, recommend vaccine

Diphtheria, *Polio*, Tetanus, recommend updating vaccines

Malaria, in most rural areas under 1980 ft. (600 m), year-round, recommend chloroquine and Fansidar prophylaxis

VIETNAM

No IAMAT doctor available; water, milk products, and cold food unsafe

Required

Yellow fever vaccine (those over age one) if from infected country previous 14 days

Risks

Cholera, recommend vaccine

Infectious hepatitis, recommend 2 cc gamma globulin

Plague, recommend vaccine or daily sulfonamides if wild rodent exposure likely

Rabies, recommend pre-exposure vaccine, avoid mammals

Typhoid, recommend vaccine

Diphtheria, Polio, Tetanus, recommend updating vaccines

Dengue, recommend anti-mosquito measures dusk to dawn

Malaria, in all areas under 1980 ft. (600 m) year-round, recommend chloroquine and Fansidar prophylaxis

VIRGIN ISLANDS (British)

No IAMAT doctor available; water probably safe but not recommended; milk products and food safe

Required

None

Risks

Diphtheria, Polio, Tetanus, recommend updating vaccines

VIRGIN ISLANDS (USA)

IAMAT doctor available; water probably safe but not recommended; milk products and food safe

Required

None

Risks

Diphtheria, Polio, Tetanus, recommend updating vaccines

WAKE ISLAND

No IAMAT doctor available; water probably safe but not recommended; incomplete data on milk products; food safe

Required

None

Risks

Diphtheria, Polio, Tetanus, recommend updating vaccines

YEMEN ARAB REPUBLIC (SANA)

No IAMAT doctor available; water, milk products, and cold food unsafe

Required

Yellow fever vaccine (those over age one) if from infected country previous 14 days

Risks

Infectious hepatitis, recommend 2 cc gamma globulin

Typhoid, recommend vaccine

Diphtheria, Polio, Tetanus, recommend updating vaccines

Malaria, most areas under 4620 ft. (1400 m) Sept.-Feb., recommend chloroquine prophylaxis

YEMEN, DEMOCRATIC REPUBLIC OF (ADEN)

415 No IAMAT doctor available; water, milk products, and cold food unsafe

Required

Yellow fever vaccine (those over age one) if from infected country previous 14 days

Risks

Cholera, recommend vaccine

Infectious hepatitis, recommend 2 cc gamma globulin

Rabies, recommend pre-exposure vaccine, avoid mammals

Typhoid, recommend vaccine

Diphtheria, *Polio*, *Tetanus*, recommend updating vaccines

Malaria, in most areas (except Aden) year-round, recommend chloroquine prophylaxis

YUGOSLAVIA

IAMAT doctor available; water probably safe but not recommended; milk products and food safe

Required

None

Risks

Diphtheria, *Polio*, *Tetanus*, recommend updating vaccines

ZAIRE

IAMAT doctor available; water, milk products, and cold food unsafe

Required

Yellow fever vaccine (those over age one) if from infected country previous 14 days or if destined for areas south of 10° S

Risks

Yellow fever, recommend vaccine

Cholera, recommend vaccine

Infectious hepatitis, recommend 2 cc gamma globulin

Plague, recommend vaccine or daily sulfonamide if wild rodent exposure likely

Typhus, recommend vaccine and good hygiene

Typhoid, recommend vaccine

Diphtheria, *Polio*, *Tetanus*, recommend updating vaccines

Malaria, all areas, year-round, recommend chloroquine prophylaxis

ZAMBIA

No IAMAT doctor available; water probably safe but not recommended; milk may be safe but not recommended; cold food unsafe

Required

Cholera vaccine and *Yellow fever vaccine* (those over age one) if from infected country previous 14 days

Risks

Cholera, recommend vaccine

Infectious hepatitis, recommend 2 cc gamma globulin

Typhus, recommend vaccine and good hygiene

Typhoid, recommend vaccine

Diphtheria, *Polio*, *Tetanus*, recommend updating vaccines

Malaria, all areas, Nov.-May, recommend chloroquine prophylaxis

ZIMBABWE (Formerly Rhodesia)

IAMAT doctor available; water probably safe but not recommended; milk products and food safe

Required

Yellow fever vaccine if from infected country previous 14 days

Risks

Infectious hepatitis, recommend 2 cc gamma globulin

Typhus, recommend vaccine and good hygiene

Typhoid, recommend vaccine

Diphtheria, *Polio*, *Tetanus*, recommend updating vaccines

Malaria, all areas, recommend chloroquine prophylaxis

IAMAT Directory to Doctors

(by City and Country)

This is the directory of IAMAT (International Association for Medical Assistance to Travellers) centers which recommend physicians to travelers. The doctors are selected by IAMAT on the basis of the following:

1. Review of professional qualifications in light of IAMAT's requirements,
2. Ability to speak English in addition to the native tongue,
3. Acceptance of the schedule fees established by IAMAT.

To use this directory, look up the name of the city. The telephone number listed is the IAMAT Center for that city. The Center will furnish you with the daily list of approved doctors (both internists and specialists in all fields of medicine), from the panel on 24-hour duty.

ARGENTINA

Buenos Aires

Hospital Britanico de Buenos Aires
Director General: Michael Lowe, MD — 231081 9
Iamat Co-ordinator:
Goodman Mercer, MD

Chaco

Santatorio Adventista Loma Linda — 280
Medical Director: Arturo J. Weiss, MD

Concepcion del Uruguay

Clinica Uruguay
Medical Director: Raul Barbara, MD
Administrative Director: A. Artusi, MD — 27 43 17 19
Iamat Co-ordinator:
Jose Angel Pons, MD

San Carlos de Bariloche

Santorio y Maternidad "Cumelen" — 222 43 247 90
Medical Director: Enrique L. Giron, MD — 247 94

ARUBA

see Netherlands Antilles

AUSTRALIA

Melbourne

St Vincent's Hospital
Iamat Co-ordinator:
E.W.R. Grace, OBE. FHA — 410 221

AUSTRIA

Alt-Aussee

Iamat Center — Puchen 231 06 152/24 88
Co-ordinator: Herbert Walter, MD

Bad Ischl

Landeskrankenhaus
Medical Director: Prim. Doz. Dr.
Richard Gmeiner 31 81
Iamat Co-ordinator: Peter Mathes, MD

Bludenz

Krankenhaus der Stadt Bludenz
Medical Director: Werner Albrich, MD 36 51 2 3
Administrative Director:
Albert Wittwer, LLD

Kitzbuehel

Iamat Center — Franz Reisch Str. 13 24 16
Co-ordinator: George Plahl, MD

Iamat Center — Erlerstrasse 1 45 94
Co-ordinator: Jeffrey Iacobucci, MD 40 15

Salzburg

Diakonissenkrankenhaus 77 581
Iamat Co-ordinator: Anton Heiser, MD

St. Anton am Arlberg

Iamat Center — The Clinic 22 33 - 24 30
Co-ordinator: Otto Murr, MD

Seefeld

Iamat Center 23 88
Co-ordinator: Bruno Genelin, MD

Vienna

Iamat Center — Graben 13 523 857
Co-ordinator: Erwin A. Mayer, MD

Rudolfiner Haus 361 250
Iamat Co-ordinators:
Erwin A. Mayer, MD
Alfred Stiskal, MD

BAHAMAS

Freeport

The Antoni Clinic — 33 333/4/5
Medical Director: Albert A. Antoni,
MDS, DDS, FRCD (C)

Iamat Center — Adventurers Way — 352 7288
Co-ordinator: Izabella E. Horsfall, MD,BS — 352 5052

BALEARIC ISLANDS

(see Spain)

BANGLADESH

Dhaka

Holy Family Hospital of Bangladesh
Red Cross Society — 283 115/7
Administrative Director: M. M. Yussouf

BELGIUM

Antwerpen

Iamat Center — Karel Oomsstraat 44 — 237 3130
Co-ordinator: Frans Van Look, MD

BOLIVIA

Cochabamba

Centro de Salud — 21 887
Iamat Co-ordinator: Rubén Gonzales, MD — 24 200

La Paz

Boston Clinic — 322 410 - 378 778
Medical Director:
Hugo Palazzi M., MD, FACS — 794 700 - 371 826

Santa Cruz

Iamat Center — 38 Suarez de Figueroa — 23 075
Co-ordinator: Percy Boland, MD, MPH

BOTSWANA

Gaborone

Iamat Center — 945 Kaunda Rd.	52 221
Co-ordinator: A. E. Bhoola, MB, BCh	71 110
Iamat Center — 4853 Independence Ave.	51 743
Co-ordinators: T. J. S. Letsunyane, BSc, MBChB	53 366
L.F. Matthews, MBChB	

Kanye

Kanye Hospital	333
Medical Director: R. F. Snide, MD	

BRAZIL

Brasilià, D.F.

Casa de Saúde Santa Lucia	243 5566
Medical Director: Edvaldo Leal, MD	
Iamat Co-ordinator: Celio Menicucci, MD	

Campo Grande

Hospital Adventista de Campo Grande	624 8571
Medical Director: João Kiefer Filho, MD	
Iamat Co-ordinator: René Gross, MD	

Fortaleza

Iamat Center — Ed. Lobras Sala 529, 5°andar	231 1014
Co-ordinator: Antônio Luis de Almeida Vale, MD	231 2610

Manaus

"Prontocord" Pronto Socorro Cardio	232 0749 - 232 0008
Iamat Co-ordinator: Juan Vila Beneyto, MD	232 0655

Pôrto Alegre

Iamat Center — Rua Silva Só, 255	314 480 - 315 483
Co-ordinator: Prof. José Martins Job, MD	318 207

Rio de Janeiro — Copacabana

Iamat Center — Av. Princesa Isabel 323, Suite 1113 — 225 3443
Co-ordinator: H. C. de Souza Araujo, Jr., MD

Rio de Janeiro — Botafogo

Iamat Center — Rua Sorocaba 464 — 226 8596 - 245 5780
Co-ordinator: Rafael Leite Luna, MD — 286 0022

Rio de Janeiro — Cosme Velho

Hospital Adventista Silvestre — 265 0212
Medical Director: Zildomar Deucher, MD — 295 0996

Salvador

Atendimentos Médicos — 245 8411 - 245 9139
Administrative Director: Jorge Cerqueira, MD — 254 9693
Technical Director: Luis Antônio Medeiros, MD

São Paulo

Hospital Samaritano — 512 154
Medical Director: Silvio Larocca de Paiva, MD
Administrative Director: José Sadyneto, MD

CAMEROON, UNITED REPUBLIC OF

Yaounde

Iamat Center — 224 523
Co-ordinator: Anne-Marie Nkoulou, MD — 220 586

CANADA

Banff — 762 2233

The Banff Clinic
Medical Director: R. W. Fleming, MD

Calgary

Iamat Center — 2303 - 4th Street S.W., 9th floor — 263 1000
Co-ordinator: S. Grunberg, MD, LMCC

Chicoutimi

Hôpital de Chicoutimi 549 2195
Medical Director: Léon Demers, MD
General Director: Maurice Cardinal

Edmonton

Edmonton General Hospital —
Emergency Dept. 482 4421
Chief Casualty Officer: G. Trepanier, MD
Supervisor, Emergency Dept.:
Mrs. T. Baril

Kamloops

Royal Inland Hospital 374 5111
Medical Director:
G. R. Davies, MD, FRCS(C)

Magog

Le Centre Hospitalier La Providence 843 3381
Medical Director: Jean-Paul Goulet, MD
Administrative Director:
M. Claude Noel

Medicine Hat

Medical Arts Building 527 2281
Medical Director: J. H. Hook, MD
Administrative Director: K. G. Gore
Iamat Co-ordinator: J. M. Cowan, MD, FRCS

Morden

Morden District General Hospital 822 4411
Medical Director: J. C. Menzies, MD
Administrative Director: O. Hamm

Quebec

The Jeffrey Hale's Hospital 683 4471
Medical Director: P. E. Kozak, MD
Administrative Director: R. Auger

L'Hôtel Dieu de Québec 694 5151
Medical Director: André Pothier, MD
Executive Director: V. G. Laurin, Eng.

Regina

Iamat Center — 950 Midtown Centre, 1783 Hamilton St.	527 4656
Co-ordinator: E. F. Abd-Elmessih, MD	586 3829

St. Albert

The Associate Medical Clinic	458 1234
Medical Director: W. Mirlin, MD	
Administrative Director: Mrs. J. Hunt	

Saint-Hyacinthe

Hôpital Honoré Mercier — Emergency Dept.	773 6811
Medical Director: Roger Lachance, MD	
Executive Director: M. Gilles Groulx	

Sault Ste. Marie

Group Health Center	949 8391
Medical Directorr: T. A. Ferrier, MD	
Administrative Director: F. H. Griffith	

Vancouver

St. Paul's Hospital — Emergency Room	682 2344
Vice President, Medical: E. John Gray, MD	

Windsor

The Metropolitan General Hospital	254 1661
Administrative Director: J. R. Hastings	

CENTRAL AFRICAN REPUBLIC

Bangui

La Clinique Docteur Chouaib	26 52
Medical Director: Raymond Chouaib, MD	
Administrative Director: J. Ayad	

CHILE

Antofagasta

Iamat Center — Prat 482	22 071
Co-ordinator: Pedro Becker Cummins, MD	21 586

Santiago

Iamat Center — Eliodero Yáñez 1049 | 494 001
Co-ordinator: E. Harold Coghlan, MD

Iamat Center — Perez Valenzuela 1686 | 744 087 - 465 809
Co-ordinator:
Alberto C. Spoerer, MD, FACC | 491 636 - 46 087

Viña del Mar

Iamat Center — Calle Valparaiso 694 | 84 873
Co-ordinator: Kenneth H. Jones, MD | Reñaca 110

CHINA (TAIWAN)

Taipei

Taiwan Adventist Hospital | 771-8151
President: Albert R. Deininger
Chief of Staff: James E. Lin, MD

COLOMBIA

Barranquilla

Iamat Center — Carrera 43, No. 41-27 | 321 769 - 325 711
Co-ordinator: Mario Zurek Mesa, MD | 343 030 - 349 073

Bogota

Clinica Marly | 278 1020 - 232 0872
Medical Director:
Jorge Cavalier Gaviria, MD | 236 1503
Iamat Co-ordinator: Bernardo
Samper, MD | 236 3296 - 254 9221

Cali

Iamat Center — Calle 26 Norte #4N-35 | 661 244 - 688 230
Co-ordinator: Carlos Kreisberger D., MD | 671 701

Hospital Universitario del Valle Evaristo
Garcia | 501 151
Medical Director: Armando González, MD

Cartagena

The Hospital Bocagrande 40 270/1/2/3 - 43 901
Medical Director:
Hernando Espinosa, MD 44 850
Administrative Director:
Antonio Guette P.

Medellin

Clínica Soma 455 600
Medical Director: Norman D. Pizano, MD

CONGO, PEOPLE'S REPUBLIC OF THE

Brazzaville

La Clinique 811 493
Medical Director: B.C.P. Denjean, MD

CURAÇAO

(see Netherlands Antilles)

CYPRUS

Nicosia

The Nicosia Clinic 77 022/3
Medical Director:
C. S. Christopoulos, MD, FRCS
Iamat Co-ordinator:
C. D. Christodoulakis, MD

DENMARK

Hellerup — Copenhagen

Iamat Center — Margrethevej 6 622 082
Co-ordinator: Ole Drucker, MD 623 708

DOMINICAN REPUBLIC

Santiago

Clinica Corominas 582 1171 - 582 2589 - 582 3913
Medical Director:
Salomón Jorge, MD, FACC, FACP

Santo Domingo

Centro Médico Nacional 682 0171 - 689 8787 - 689 1565
Iamat Co-ordinators: Fernándo Ariza Mendoza, MD
José H. Ornes, MD

ECUADOR

Guayaquil

Iamat Center — 821 Boyacá St.	301 785
Co-ordinator: Angel Serrano, MD, FACS, FICS	301 373
Institutio de Cardiologia — 202 Hurtado St.	516 879
Iamat Co-ordinator: Gilberto R. Peñafiel, MD	525 267

Libertad-Salinas

Iamat Center — Calle 9 de Octubre 455	141
Co-ordinator: Luís Celleri A., MD	

Quito

Clínica Americana	234 471 - 236 942
Iamat Co-ordinators: Waldo W. Stiles, MD	
Jacinto Alvarado, MD	234 117

EGYPT

Cairo

Iamat Center — 11 Emad el Din St.	910 816
Co-ordinator: Samir B. Bassily, MD	916 424
Iamat Center — 87, Road 9, Maadi	633 105
Co-ordinator: Sherif Doss, MB, MSc	634 085

EL SALVADOR

San Salvador

Clinical Médicas	25 0277 Ext. 178 or 167
Medical Director: Prof. Juán José Fernández	25 8325
Director of Clinical Pathology: Max Bloch, MD	22 2809

Ed. Medico Dental — 1ª Calle Pte,
19 Ave. N. 224 941 - 217 820
Iamat Co-ordinator:
Luis J. Escalante, MD, MRCP 230 609

FINLAND

Helsinki

Iamat Center — Bulevardi 10 A 640 604
Co-ordinator: Stefan Barner-Rasmussen, MD 427 283

FRANCE

Aix en Provence

Iamat Center — 19 bis, Avenue des
Belges 263 311
Co-ordinator: Yves Lemière, MD

Clinique du Parc Rambot 261 447
Medical Director: G. L. Cartotto, MD
Iamat Co-ordinators: Yves Lemière, MD
A. Leoncini, MD

Antibes

"Le Sylvana" — 72, Bd. Wilson 615 089 - 344 730
Iamat Co-ordinators: Jacques de Saint-
Martin, MD 614 353
Claude Gobin, MD 651 031

Biarritz

Iamat Center — 7, avenue de la Reine
Victora 241 010
Co-ordinator: R. Ducoudré, MD

Cannes

Iamat Center — 75, rue d'Antibes 393 028
Co-ordinator: Pierre Guillemin, MD

Chartres

Clinique Chirurgicale Saint-François 215 285
Medical Director:
Jean-Paul de Fourmestraux, MD

Dijon

Clinique Médico-Chirurgicale — 413 812 - 413 171
Medical Director: Louis Parodi, MD
Administrative Director: A. Foin

Frejus

Clinique des Lauriers — 512 280
Medical Director: J. P. Lavernhe, MD
Administrative Director: R. Lavernhe, MD

Juan-Les-Pins

Clinique Wilson — 615 089 - 344 730
Iamat Co-ordinators: Jacques de Saint-Martin, MD
Claude Gobin, MD

La Rochelle

Iamat Center — Place Charles Fromentin, Cours Forbin — 425 162
Co-ordinator: E. A. Jousselin, MD — 421 922 - 425 350

Le Cannet

Iamat Center — 10, rue Henri Germain — 454 992
Co-ordinator: Daniel Beddouk, MD

Le Havre

Iamat Center — 9, rue Romain-Rolland — 460 298
Co-ordinator: Pierre Barthès, MD

Limoges

Iamat Center — 11 Place Franklin D. Roosevelt — 346 186
Co-ordinator: Jacques Lamoure, MD

Lourdes

Iamat Center — 3 Place du Marcadal — 940 792
Co-ordinator: Jean Maur, MD

Lyon

Hôpital Ed. Herriot — 548 191
Medical Director: Prof. J. Traeger, MD

Marseille

Clinique de la Résidence du Parc | 759 191
Medical Directors: Vincent Pol, MD
Prof. R. Courbier, MD
Norbert Boineau, MD

Nancy

Iamat Center — Centre de Montet
Octroi | 552 796
Co-ordinator: Henri Claude Person, MD

Nantes

Iamat Center — 24, rue du Calvaire | (40) 482 336
Co-ordinator: Yves M. George, MD

Nice

Iamat Center — 47 ter, rue du
Maréchal-Joffre | 886-079
Co-ordinator: G. Guillermond, MD

Iamat Center — 14, rue d'Alsace-
Lorraine | 886 164
Co-ordinator: Jean Ducoeur, MD | 814 965

Iamat Center — 3, rue Cronstadt | 881 426
Co-ordinator: Jacquues Gabay, MD

Iamat Center — 35, Boulevard Victor
Hugo | 884 214
Co-ordinator: Georges Ch. Thooris, MD

Orly

Clinique Chirurgicale d'Athis-Mons | 904 5080
Medical Director: A. Elmadeli, MD | 938 4528
Iamat Co-ordinator: Jean Connault, MD | 938 4805

Paris

The American Hospital of Paris | 637 7200
63, Boulevard Victor Hugo, Neuilly-sur-Seine

(Nonmember but cooperating hospital, not pledged to rate schedule.)

Saint Jean de Luz

Polyclinique — 262 140 - 260 247
Medical Director: Paul Badiola, MD

Strasbourg

Hôpital Civil — Pavillon Leriche — 367 111 Ext. 3226
Iamat Co-ordinator: Prof. F. Stephan, MD

Iamat Center — 1, Ave. du General de Gaulle — 600 723
Co-ordinator: Roland Abib, MD

Toulouse

Iamat Center — 1, rue Languedoc — 527 002
Co-ordinator: Jean Delprat, MD — 817 879

Tours

Iamat Center —58, rue du Cluzel — 054 629
Co-ordinator: Gérard Kahn, MD

Vichy

Iamat Center — 4, rue d'Italie — 983 599
Co-ordinator: P.-C. Stavré, MD

FRENCH GUIANA

Cayenne

Iamat Center — 38, rue Lieutenant Brassé — 310 464
Co-ordinator: Henri Henriot, MD

GABON

Lambarene

The Albert Schweitzer Hospital
Medical Director: A. K. Steiner, MD
Administrative Director: Max Caulet

GERMANY, FEDERAL REPUBLIC OF

Berlin (West)

Iamat Center — Medical Center, Berlin
Penta Hotel, Nuernbergerstrasse 65 — 240 011
Medical Director: Wilhelm Engert, MD

Bonn

Medizinische Universitaetsklinik — 192 256
Medical Director: Prof. A. W. v. Eiff, MD

Bremen

Iamat Center — Holler Allee 5 — 343 488
Co-ordinator: E. Georg Brautlecht, MD

Düsseldorf

Iamat Center — Niederrheinstrasse 224a — 452 272
Co-ordinator: Hans Max Poszich, MD — 432 757

Düsseldorf — Grafenberg

Iamat Center — Geibelstrasse 45 — 663 444
Co-ordinator: Helmut Heilborn, MD

Düsseldorf - Oberkassel

Iamat Center — Adalbertstrasse 4 — 571 950
Co-ordinator: Gerd Engstfeld, MD

Freiburg

Iamat Center — Turnseestrasse 6 — 74 431 - 82 395
Co-ordinators: Max Bass, MD
Gideon Bass, MD

Giessen

Iamat Center — An der Johanneskirche 2 — 73 232
Co-ordinator: Hans Ludwig Althaus, MD

Heidelberg

Medizinische Universitaetsklinik — 532 391
Ludolf-Krehl-Klinik
Medical Director: Prof. G. Schettler, MD

Karlsruhe/Durlach

Iamat Center — Badener Str. 1 — 41 171
Co-ordinator: Wolfgang Hesse, MD

Koblenz

Iamat Center — Rheinstrasse 28 — 32 166
Co-ordinator: Karl Gassen, MD

Leutkirch

Iamat Center — 23 Untere Grabenstrasse — (07) 561 2200
Co-ordinator: Eyck Fintelmann, MD, FAAOO — 561 2207

Mannheim

Mannheim Uni-Klinikum — 28 604
Medical Director: Prof. O. Hallen, MD
Administrative Director: R. Decker, dipl.Kfm.
Iamat Co-ordinator: Prof. Peter Stoll, MD, FIAC

Munich

Iamat Center — Gruenwalderstrasse 53 — 692 7672
Co-ordinator: Ernst Pfister, MD

Nürnberg

Iamat Center — Hallerhüttenstrasse 5 — 468 115
Co-ordinator: G. Antonopoulos, MD

Oberammergau

Iamat Center — In der Furch 3 — 47 55
Co-ordinator: Franz Kreuter, MD

Pforzheim

Iamat Center — Kiehnlestrasse 15 — 12 028
Co-ordinator: Karl W. Hayler, MD

GHANA

Accra

Tudu Clinic — 24 833
Medical Director: A. A. Skiwumi, MB, CHB, MRCP (Edin.), DTM and H (L'pool)

GREECE

Athens

Iamat Center — Ilisia-Hilton	721 1681
3 Vrasida Street	672 1514
Co-ordinator: Paris Raftopoulos, MBBCH (Rand), FCPSA	682 7940
Hemodialysis Center — Vasilisis Sofias 60	791 976
Medical Director: Steven E. Magiorakos, MD	720 210

Athens - Kolonaki

Iamat Center — 26 Karneadou St.	721 0200
Co-ordinator: Vasilis A. Georgiou, MD	

Corfou

Saint Spiridion General Clinic	37 284
Iamat Co-ordinator: Spyros Chryssikopulos, MD	

Halkis

Skianis Polyclinic	24 522
Medical Directors: George Skianis, MD John Skianis, MD	

Ioannina

St. Anaryiri Clinic	23 991 - 23 992 - 23 994
Medical Directors: J. Baltoyannis, MD S. Baltoyannis, MD	

Kavala

General Hospital "Blue Cross of Kavala"	228 882 - 228 651
Iamat Co-ordinator: Dimitrios I. Asteriadis, MD, FICS	

Rhodes

General Hospital of Rhodes	25 555
General Director: Kalamatar Simeou	
Iamat Co-ordinator: John Sotiriou, MD	29 333

GUADELOUPE

Pointe-a-Pitre

Clinique St. Nicolas	821 966
Iamat Co-ordinator: Georges Nithila, MD	820 166

GUATEMALA

Guatemala

Hospital Herrera Llerandi	66 771/2/3/4/5

Administrative Director: Roberto Eichenberger, MD
Iamat Co-ordinators:
Rodolfo Herrera Llerandi, MD
Mario Duarte, MD
Carlos Pérez Avendaño, MD

GUYANA

Georgetown

St. Joseph Mercy Hospital	72 070 - 72 079

Consultant Physician: Hughley H. Hanoman, MB, BCh, DTM&H, MRCGP, MRCP
Administrative Director:
Sister Mary Admirabilis, RSM

HAITI

Port-Au-Prince

Centre Médicale	23 429 - 24 023

Medical Director: Alix Adams, MD, FICS
Administrative Director:
Grégoire Cherubin

Hôpital du Canapé Vert	21 052 - 21 053

Medical Director: A. Miot, MD

HONDURAS

Tegucigalpa

Hospital Viera and Clinicas Viera — 223 156/7/8/9
Medical Directors:
Juan Andonie Fernández, MD
Edgardo Alonso Medina, MD

HONG KONG

Hong Kong

Sing Tao Medical Centre — 33 Queen's Road, Central — 5-266 505
Iamat Co-ordinators:
Jean Woo, MB BChir, MRCP (UK) — 5-258 158
Wai-Ming Chen, MD, MCPS(C) — 5-735 902
C. M. Wong, MD FRCR, DMRD
After office hours call: 3-314 341, page Dr. C. M. Wong No. 2886

(Patients calling from Hong Kong side need not dial prefix 5: patients calling from Kowloon need not dial prefix 3).

HUNGARY

Budapest

Postgraduate Medical School — 290 265 - 165 131
IV Dept. of Internal Medicine — 355 082
Iamat Co-ordinator: Prof. E. Szatloczky, MD

ICELAND

Reykjavik

St. Joseph's Hospital — 19 600
Medical Director: Bjarni Jonsson, MD
Administrative Director: Sister Marie Hildegardis

INDIA

Agra

Jaggi Nursing & Maternity Home — 73 315 - 75 516
Medical Directors:
R. K. Jaggi, MB BS, FAGS
Nita Jaggi, MB, BS, DGO

Malhotra Nursing & Maternity Home — 73 446
Medical Directors:
R. M. Malhotra, BSc, MIBBS, FICS
Prabha Malhotra, MBBS, DGO

Ahmedabad

Heart Foundation and Research Institute
Heart Care Clinic — C-11, Silver Arc, Gujarat College — 78 999
Medical Directors:
Sumant M. Shah, MD, MRCP, FCCP, FICA — 444 201
Nitin S. Shah, MD, FRSM, HRFKCH, HRFHH (Lond) — 388 450, 444 181

Bangalore

St. Philomena's Hospital — 57 046 - 54 061
Medical Director:
C. D. Jacob, MD, BSc, MBBS, MRCP

Bareilly

Clara Swain Hospital — 31 11 - 32 47
Medical Director: A. Inder Shaw, MD
Administrative Director: Y. M. Nilajgi

Bombay

Iamat Center — Shanti Kuteer,
N. Subhas Rd., Nariman Point — 241 025
Co-ordinator: R. H. Dastur, MD — 240 026 - 825 638

The Breach Candy Hospital — 363 651
Medical Director: Jal Dubash, MD (Lond.), FRP (Lond.)
Administrative Director: P. S. Kaicker

Calcutta

Belle Vue Clinic 442 321
Chief Cardiologist:
K. B. Baksi, MD, Dip. Card. (Cal.)
Administrative Director: B. L. Gupta

Woodlands Nursing Home 453 951
(The East India Clinic)
Medical Director and Secretary:
B. B. Guha Thakurta, MD, FRCP, MRCP, DTM&H, DGO

Indore

Pushp-Kuni Hospital 55 23 - 63 13
Medical Director:
Chamanlal Nagrath, LRCP (Lond.), MRCS (Eng.), FRCS (Engl.)

Jaipur-Rajasthan

S.D.M. Hospital and Zoraster Poly Clinic 74 149
Raja Park Nursing Home
Senior Consultant:
Hans Kumar, MBBS, MAMS, DTD, FACS
General Surgeon: Vijay Sikka, MBBS, MS
Obstetrician: Usha Sikka, MBBS, MD

Kodarma-Bihar

Holy Family Hospital 29

Ludhiana

The Christian Medical College and Hospital 29 06 - 25 06
Medical Director:
K. N. Nambudripad, FRCA (Ed.) MS
Administrative Director: John D. Rollins

Madras

Lady Willingdon Nursing Home 85 868 - 86 893 - 86 676
Medical Director: B. Krishna Rau, MS, FRCS (Edin), FRCA (Eng.)

Heart and Lung Clinic, H.M. Hospital 72,236 - 74 166
Medical Director:
Prathap C. Reddy, MB, FCCP, FICA

New Dehli

Holy Family Hospital	632 355 - 632 383 - 632 444
Iamat Co-ordinators:	
B. B. Mathur, MD	635 353
S. K. Sridharan, MD	668 333
S. Mukherji, MD	667 759

Nuzvid-Krishna

Andhra Pradesh	
Giffard Memorial Hosital	30

Ottappalam

Seventh-day Adventist Hospital	201

Medical Director: K. P. George, MS
Iamat Co-ordinator:
Mary Lucile Small MD, FACOG

Patna-Bihar

Kurji Holy Family Hospital	23 536 - 22 136

Poona

Poona Adventist Medical Centre	449 726 - 28 656

Medical Director:
C. A. Ninan, FRCS, FICS

Simla

Simla Sanitarium and Hospital	28 04 - 56 79

Medical Director:
B. Y. Bazliel, MRCOG, MBChB, LRCP, MRCS

Tuticorin

Sacred Heart Hospital	704

Medical Director: M. Krishna Nair, MD
Administrative Director:
Mother M. Elisabeth
Administrator in Charge:
Sister Paula Graf

INDONESIA

Jakarta

Iamat Center — Jalan Singamangaraja 51 — 771 445 - 744 004
Co-ordinator: Karnen Baratawidjaja, MD
Internist and Allergy Consultant

Jogjakarta

Bethesda Hospital (Rumah Sakit "Bethesda") — 22 81/2
General Director: Guuno Samekto, MD
Medical Director:
Lukas Budi Gunawan, MD
Administrative Director:
R. Rachman, MECSC

Kediri

Kediri Baptist Hospital (Rumah Sakit Baptis) — 21 170 - 41 172
Medical Director: Donald Duvall, MD
Administrative Director: Frank Tan

Surabaya

Iamat Center — 100 Jalan Dinoyo — 67 722 - 60 985
Co-ordinator: Tjiptono Darmadji, MD

IRELAND, NORTHERN

Belfast

Iamat Center — 344 Antrim Rd. — 776 600
Co-ordinator: Patrick T. McGeough — 777 759

Iamat Center — 279 Antrim Rd. — 745 157
Co-ordinator: Eugene Maguire — 771 864

IRELAND, REPUBLIC OF

Dublin

Iamat Centeer — 11 Proby Square, Blackrock — 882 683
Co-ordinator: John F. Fleetwood, MD — 972 727

Iamat Center — 54 Woodbine Rd., Blackrock 691 581
Co-ordinator: W. A. Ryan, FRCPI, MRCGP

ISRAEL

Ashdod

Iamat Center — Rehov Haalmogim 41 (055) 42 944
Co-ordinatorr: Alan Levine, MD

Ashkelon (Afridar)

Iamat Center — 6 Hadrorstreet 33 396
Co-ordinator: U. van Dam, MD

Iamat Center — 22 Rehov Hatamar 28 926
Co-ordinator: A. Hurwitz, MD

Beer-Sheba

Soroka Medical Center 77 111
Iamat Co-ordinator:
M. R. Quastel, MD, PhD 74 817

Eilat

Josephtal Hospital 23 01 - 31 51
Head of Medical Department:
Edward Hardoon, MD

Haifa (Mount Carmel)

Elisha Hospital 81 418/9

Jerusalem

Hadassah University Hospital 411 111
Director General: K. J. Mann, MD
Deputy Director General: Jack Karpas, MD
(Only for out-patient, casualty service and hospital admission: not for home or hotel calls. Specialist private consultation clinics on the hospital premises only.)

Iamat Center — 9 Shlomo Molcho Street
Co-ordinators:
Prof. Eli Davis, MD, MSc, FRCP
B. Kaplan, MD
For office consultations: 633 712
For hotel and home calls: 526 928

Natanya

Iamat Center — 37 Jerusalem Street 22 930
Co-ordinators: Joshua Nafte, MBBCh 24 735
I. A. Zuckerbrod, MB, ChB 40 140
S. Kugler, MD 35 022

Nazareth

Iamat Center — 11/206 Nazareth 71 360
Co-ordinator: Aziz S. Srouji, MD

Savyon

Iamat Center — 15 Hatichon Street 756 688
Co-ordinator: Joseph Book, MD, FACS

Tel Aviv

Iamat Center (03) 756 688
Co-ordinator: Joseph Book, MD, FACS

Assutah Hospital 245 211 - 240 697
Medical Director: B. Frishman, MD

ITALY

Alassio

Casa di Cura Villa Paradiso 40 456
Iamat Co-ordinator: Prof. Ignazio Abbo, MD

Albenga

Casa di Cura S. Michele 51 494 - 51 495
Medical Director: Prof. Libero Nante, MD
Administrative Director:
Mrs. Maria Rosa Nante

Bolzano

Iamat Center — Medical Building, 8 Via
Cassa Di Risparmio
Co-ordinator: Germar Schick, MD 39 342 - 41 384

Carate Brianza

Clinica Zucchi 902 801
General Director: Antonio Frova, MD
Medical Director: Piero Pirola, MD

Feltre

Casa di Cura Villabruna Bellati 800 41
Medical Director: Giovanni Russo, MD
Administrative Director: Francesco Villabruna

Florence

Iamat Center — Via della Scala 35/A
Co-ordinator: Enrico de Santi, MD 202 0263 - 212 010

Casa di Cura "Piccola Compagnia di Maria" 572 556/7/8
Medical Director: G. Ferrari, MD
Iamat Co-ordinators:
Enrico de Santi, MD 202 0263 - 212 010
Salvo Mori, MD 681 3319 - 576 423
(Nonmember but cooperating hospital not pledged to rate schedule.)

Latina

General Hospital S. Maria Goretti 499 911
Medical Director: Prof. Renato Busco, MD
Administrative Director: Serafino Scarpelli

Macerata

Ospedale Generale Provinciale 20 83
Medical Director: Prof. Luigi Salatucci, MD

Merano

The Kneringer Clinic 22 480
Medical Director: Josef Unterhuber, MD
Administrative Director: Pietro Piva

Messina

Istituto Ortopedico Del Mezzogiorno d'Italia 812 881/2/3
Medical Director:
Prof. Franco Scalabrino, MD 811 509
Administrative Director:
Antonio Di Pasquale

Monza

Clinica Zucchi 389 451/2/3/5
General Director: Antonio Frova, MD
Medical Director: Giulio Dorigotti, MD

Naples

The International Hospital 680 606 - 682 295 - 663 116
Medical Director: Hanna Koller, MD

Palermo

Ospedale Civico 228 200 - 592 242
Iamat Co-ordinator: Louis Joseph Pepe, MD 572 540

Perugia

Istituto di Semeiotica Medica Policlinico
Monteluce 22 905
Iamat Co-ordinator: Luigi Corea, MD 752 013

Iamat Center — Via Alessi, 19 66 209
Co-ordinator: Vito Giuliani, MD

Praia-a-Mare (Cosenza)

Ospedale Civile 0985/72 485 - 72 552
Medical Director: Serafino Molinaro, MD 2984/38 185

Rapallo

Villa Chiara Hospital 54 547 - 50 059
Medical Director: G. Bacigalupo, MD 50 677

Riccione

Iamat Center — Viale Martinelli 14 41 029
Co-ordinator: Emilio Rinaldi, MD

Rome

American Medical Center 464 143 - 485 706 - 475 7221
Medical Director: Frank Silvestri, MD 390 217
Iamat Co-ordinator: Francis Spelar, MD 878 598

Iamat Center — 11 Via Sabazio 860 502
Co-ordinator: Lucio Sannino, MD 852 154

Iamat Center — Via Senofane 230 609 1156
Co-ordinator: Renato Lungarotti, MD

San Remo

Ospedale Civile 79 921
Iamat Co-ordinator:
Prof. Giovanni Galli, MD

Siracusa

Ospedale Generale Provincale
Umberto I° 24 880 - 92 962
Medical Director:
Prof. Guido Amedoro, MD
Iamat Co-ordinator: Edoardo Ferrarini, MD

Taormina

Ospedale Civile San Vincenzo 34 50 - 34 40
Medical Director: A. Passalacqua, MD
Iamat Co-ordinator: Nicolò Garipoli, MD

Trieste

Iamat Center — Viale Miramare 23 418 608
Co-ordinator: Sergio Guastalla, MD

Turin

Clinica Pinna Pintor 590 404/503 822/595 278/599 050
Medical Director: Prof. P. Pinna Pintor, MD

Venice

Iamat Center — S. Marco Fond, ta delle
Ostreghe 2337 21 370
Co-ordinator: Salvatore Saccardo, MD

Vibo Valentia

Clinica Villa dei Gerani 41 481 - 41 476
Medical Director:
Prof. Alfredo Scermino, MD

Viterbo

Iamat Center — Corso Italia 100 33 051
Co-orrdinator: Augusto Vergati, MD

IVORY COAST

Abidjan

Le Centre Médico-Chirurgical 321 526 - 225 198
Medical Director: Georges Moreau, MD

JAMAICA

Kingston

Iamat Center — 12 Hope Road — 926 6261
Co-ordinator: George P. Provan, MD — 927 8069

Ochos Rios

Iamat Center — Park Avenue
(St. Ann's Bay) — 0972 2296 - 0972 2396
Co-ordinator: Noel A. Black, MD

Port Antonio

The Port Antonio General Hospital — 993 2646
Medical Director: Neville M. Antonio, MD

St. Ann's Bay

Iamat Center — Park Avenue — 22 96 - 23 96
Co-ordinator: Noel A. Black, MD

JAPAN

Hiroshima

Harada Hospital — 323 351
Medical Director: Tomin Harada, MD — 318 312

Kobe

Kobe Kaisei Hospital — 871 5201/5
Medical Director: Sister Y. Neerdaels, MD

Kyoto

Sakabe Clinic — 231 1624
Medical Director: Yoshio Sakabe, MD

Naha-Okinawa

Adventist Medical Center — 331 107
Medical Director: James R. Wood, MD

Osaka

Yodogawa Christian Hospital — 322 2250
Superintendent: Frank A. Brown, Jr., MD
(not for hotel or home calls)

Tokyo

Tokyo Sanitarium-Hospital — 392 6151
Medical Director: Takaharu Hayashi, MD
Administrative Director: Toshio Takahara
Iamat Co-ordinator:
C. Delmar Johnson, MD, FACS

Yokohama

Bluff Hospital — 641 6961
Medical Director: Koichi Fujii, MD, FACS

JORDAN

Amman

The Palestine Hospital — 64 171 - 63 918 - 62 976
Medical Director:
Sami Khoury, MD, FICS, FACS FRCS

KENYA

Mombasa

Iamat Center — City House, Nyerere Avenue — 25 824/5
Co-ordinators: G. A. B. Cunningham, MD, FRCGP, DRCOG, DIH
J. B. O. Okanga, MRCP
P. J. Nicklin, MBBS, DA

Katherine Bibby Hospital — 24 191/2/3
Chairman Medical Board: G. A. B. Cunningham, MD, FRCGP, DRCOG, DIH

Nairobi

Iamat Center — Electricity House, Harambee Avenue — 20 832 - 26 253
Co-ordinators:
Clara D. Cruz, BSc, MBBCh — 61 563
Manuel J. D'Cruz, MB, FRCS, DLO

Iamat Center — Jubilee Insurance House, Wabera Street — 61 481 - 22 513
Co-ordinator:
Vera Somen, MBBS, LRCP, MRCS, MRCGP

Iamat Center — Bruce House, Standard Street 21 741
Co-ordinator: C. S. Sheth, MD

In Nairobi,

Iamat members contemplating a safari in East Africa may obtain a tourist membership (fee $3.50) from the Flying Doctors' Society of Africa which offers ambulance flights in emergencies:

The Flying Doctors' Society of Africa 27 281
Chairman: Mrs. Maddie De Mott

KOREA, REPUBLIC OF

Pusan

Wallace Memorial Baptist Hospital 430 201/2/3/4
Medical Director: Charles G. Tabor, MD 439 506/7/8
Administrative Director: Charles Wiggs

Seoul

Kangnam St. Mary's Hospital 593 9121 Ext. 121
Catholic Medical Center
Iamat Co-ordinator:
Prof. Byong Sok Min, MD 388 0477
Dept. of Internal Medicine

KUWAIT

Kuwait

Mowasat Hospital 611 536 - 611 540
Medical Director:
Wajdi Kanan, MB, ChB, FRCP, DPhil (Oxon)
Administrative Director: Maurice Tanas

LEBANON

Beirut

American University of Beirut Hospital 340 460

LESOTHO

Maseru

Iamat Center — 204 Maseru West Co-ordinator: Strong Thabo Makenete, MD	22 92 - 22 93

LIBERIA

Monrovia

The Cooper Clinic Medical Director: Henry Nehemiah Cooper, MD, FACS	261 707

LIBYAN ARAB JAMAHIRIYA

Tripoli

Iamat Center — 26, Calcutta St. Co-ordinator: Ahmad Bishti, MD	34 367 - 33 005 38 801

LIECHTENSTEIN

Schaan

Iamat Center — Landstrasse 97 Co-ordinator: Arthur Ospelt, MD	21 122 - 22 119

LUXEMBOURG

Echternach

Iamat Center — 38, rue des Remparts Co-ordinator: Georges Arnold, MD	72 237

Luxembourg

Clinique Ste. Thérèse Medical Director: Ch. Mouton, MD Iamat Co-ordinator: Raymond Schaus, MD, MRCP (Lond.)	488 181

MACAO

Macao

Iamat Center — 1-A Travessa de San Domingos 25 90
Co-ordinator: L. C. Chiu, MD

MADEIRA

(see Portugal)

MALAWI

Blantyre

Adventist Health Centre 36 999
Medical Director: L. D. Kattenhorn, MD

Lilongwe

Iamat Center — Kamuzu Procession Rd. 21 88
Co-ordinator: Ahmed I. Kharodia, MB, BS 22 21

Limbe

Iamat Center — Chirimba — Chileka Rd. 50 933
Co-ordinator: A. C. M. Bijl, MD 30 594

MALAYSIA

Georgetown — Penang

Penang Adventist Hospital 24 134
Medical Director: Sam Ketting, MD, FICS

Ipoh-Perak

Our Lady's Hospital 21 55/6
Medical Director: A. W. E. Moreira, LMS (Sing.), TDD (Wales), MD

Kota Kinabalu — Sabah

Sabah Clinic 54 190 - 33 355
Medical Director: R. B. Barrow, MS, BS, LRCP, DRCOG (London)

Kuala Lumpur

Kelinik Goh — Sungei Wang Plaza, Jalan Sultan Ismail	423 773
Medical Director: Goh Tuck Keong, MD	

Malacca

Wong Clinic — 80, Newcome Rd.	29 19
Medical Director: Wong Kong Meng, MD, MBBS	22 99

MALTA

Msida

Iamat Center — Dar il-Hena, New Str.	32 739
Co-ordinator: Robert Naudi, MD	

Sliema

Iamat Center — 26, Victoria Ave.	32 959
Co-ordinator: Cecil T. Paris, MD, BPharm.	30 376

MARTINIQUE

Fort-de-France

Centre Hospitalier — Cardiology Dept.	715 822 Ext. 204
Iamat Co-ordinator: Yves Donatien, MD	714 467
Iamat Center — 33, rue Lamartine	716 502
Co-ordinator: Raymond Rosenfeld, MD	

MAURITANIA

Nouadhibou

Polyclinic de Cansado	Cansado 837
Medical Director: Vincent E. Baqué, MD, FICS	Cansado 774
Administrative Director: J. L. Foata	

MEXICO

Chihuahua

Hospital Centro Médico — 28 332
Medical Director: Edgardo Gracia Oléa, MD
Administrative Director:
Julio Ornelas K., MD

Ciudad Juarez

Clínica Juarez — S. de R. L. de C. V. — 36 665 - 36 877
Hospital Latinoamericano, S.A.
Medical Director: Ramón Rios Ramirez, MD
Administrative Director:
Joaquín Esquivel Rosado, MD

Cuernavaca

The Red Cross and Henri Dunant
Hospital — 53 555
Medical Director:
Oscar López Cienfuegos
Administrative Director:
José I. Perez-Palma y de O.

Durango

Iamat Center — Hidalgo #139 Sur — 12 209 - 12 918
Co-ordinator: Héctor Corral, MD

Garza García

Iamat Center — Rio Colorado
203-A Ote. — 562 550 - 744 050 Ext. 501
Co-ordinator:
Bernardo Coindreau Farias, MD — 562 252 - 564 840

Guadalajara — Jalisco

Iamat Center — Pavo 112, Despacho 14 — 142 091
Co-ordinator: Eduardo Contreras Reyna, MD — 150 713

Iamat Center — Tarasco 3514 - 101, — 220 420
Ricondada Sta. Rita — 220 390
Co-ordinator:
J. Jaime Ramirez Parra, MD, FACP — 220 429

Iamat Center — 870 P. Buzeta — 414 353
Co-ordinator: Alberto Solano, MD — 232 098

Hospital Mexico Americano	413 141
Medical Director:	
José González Alonso, MD	
Administrative Director:	
Jorge Angel Rodriguez	

Hermosillo

Hospital y Clínica Sonora	34 216/7
Medical Director:	
Marco A. Mosqueira Matute, MD	38 845
Administrative Director:	
J. Jesús Preciado Morales	

Leon

Centro Médico del Bajio	36 373
Iamat Co-ordinator:	
J. Jesús Navarro Duran, MD	

Mazatlan — Sinaloa

Clinica Mazatlan	12 917 - 14 927
Medical Director:	
Gilberto Robles Guevara, MD	
Administrative Director: R. Ocampo, MD	

Merida — Yucatan

Iamat Center — Calle 57, #471	11 896 - 50 707
Co-ordinator: A. H. Puga Navarrete, MD	14 819
Iamat Center — Calle 55, #512	12 577
Co-ordinator: Ernesto Guzmán E, MD	14 024

Mexico City

Iamat Center — Paseo de las Palmas	
745, No. 402	520 3132
Co-ordinator: Prof. Francisco Biagi, MD	524 9640
The American British Cowdray Hospital	277 5000
(Nonmember but cooperating hospital, not pledged to rate schedule.)	

Monterrey — Nuevo Leon

Hospital José A. Muguerza	460 100 - 463 460
Medical Director:	
Federico Padilla Muguerza, MD	
Administrative Director:	
António Sarre	

Nogales

Central Médica De Especialidades — 20 168
Medical Director: Oscar Rojas, MD
Iamat Co-ordinator: Nadir Zeinun, MD

Oaxaca

Clinica Hospital del Carmmen — 62 612 - 66 202 - 62 238
Medical Directors:
Horacio Tenorio Sandoval, MD — 61 151
Luciano Tenorio Sandoval, MD

Pachuca

Sanatorio "Dr. Atanasio Garza Ríos" — 23 035 - 22 236/7
Medical Director:
Ignazio Gómez Tellez, MD

Puebla

Fundación Hospital Latino Americano — 424 620
Medical Director: Teofilo Treviño H., MD
General Director: Feland L. Meadows, MD
Dept. of Internal Medicine:
Enrique Montejano, MD

Puerto Vallarta — Jalisco

Iamat Center — Corona 224 — 21 305
Co-ordinator:
António Sahagún Rodriguez, MD

Queretaro

Sanatorio Dr. Núñez, Lara, MD — 21 192 - 20 161
Medical Director: Felípe Núñez Lara, MD

San Luis Potosi

Clínica de Cardiologia y Medicina Interna — day: 26 075
Medical Director:
António Rodríguez-Alvarez, MD, FACC — night: 21 901
Administrative Director:
Alicia Briones de Rodríguez

Santa Ana — Sonora

Clínica Dr. Díaz Garzón — 67
Medical Director: Juvenal Díaz Garzón, MD

Tapachula — Chiapas

Central Médico Quirurgica 62 434 - 63 701 - 51 717
Medical Director:
Juán Valdivieso Chacón, MD
Administrative Director:
Didier Cruz Fuentevilla

Taxco

Iamat Center — 2a, de Cenaobscuras #6 20 567
Co-ordinator: Clemente García Torres, MD

Torreon — Coahuila

Clínica de Diagnostico 31 415
Medical Director:
António Betancourt F., MD

Villahermosa — Tabisco

Iamat Center — Cuauhtemoc #299 20 573 - 23 010
Co-ordinator:
Manuel Rodríguez G., MD, FACS

MONACO

Monte Carlo

Iamat Center — "Europa" Residence,
Place des Moulins 506 615
Co-ordinator: Jean-Joseph Pastor, MD 309 844

Iamat Center — 14, boulevard des
Moulins 506 747
Co-ordinator: Odette Fissore, MD

Centre Hospitalier Princesse Grace 504 855
Administrative Director:
Maurice Gaziello
Iamat Co-ordinator: Odette Fissore, MD 506 747

MOROCCO

Rabat

Clinique Beauséjour 38 667/7 - 38 679
Medical Director: A. Moystad, MD
Iamat Co-ordinator: Abdeslam Tazi, MD

La Clinique de la Tour Hassan 22 906 - 25 306 - 253 06
Medical Director: Prof. Taya Alami, MD

Tanger

Iamat Center — 40 Marshan 35 943 - 35 344
Co-ordinator: George W. F. Anderson, MD

Clinique California 38 824 - 38 722
Medical Director: A. Leonetti, MD
Administrative Director:
Mrs. M. L. Salaun

NEPAL

Kathmandu

Shanta Bhawan United Mission Hospital 21 034
Medical Director:
M. G. Eldridge, MBBS, FRGOG 21 553

NETHERLANDS

Amsterdam

Iamat Center — Churchill Laan 43 642 197 - 642 111
Co-ordinator: Th. G. J. Stokman, MD

The Hague

Bronovo Hospital 264 141
Medical Director: J. E. Mellink, MD
Administrative Director: S. A. Trommel

NETHERLANDS ANTILLES
Aruba

Oranjestad

Dr. Horacio Oduber Hospital 43 00
Medical Director: F. Hage, MD

Curaçao

Willemstad

St. Elisabeth Hospital 25 100 - 24 900
Medical Director: I. R. A. Asjes, MD
Director of Nursing: R. A. Rosario

NEW HEBRIDES

Santo — Espíritu Santo Island

Aore Seventh-day Adventist Hospital

NEW ZEALAND

Christchurch

Papanui Medical Center — 529 053 - 528 006
Iamat Co-ordinator: Larry W. Skiba, MD

Wellington

Iamat Center — 161 Willis St. — 849 675 - 862 124
Co-ordinator: Harold Haydon Gray, MD

Iamat Center — 16 The Terrace — 42 219 - 759 216
Co-ordinator: Geoffrey Bruce Kiddle, MD

NIGER

Niamey

Hôpital Général — 25 21/2/3
Medical Director: Hamadou Ousseini, MD
Administrative Director: Issaka Karimou

NIGERIA

Ibadan

Oke-Ado Hospital — 23 145
Medical Director: T. O. na Oruwariye, MB BS (Lond.), FMC (G.P.)

Ilesha

Wesley Guild Hospital — Ilesha 21 16 - 21 77

Kaduna

Lafiya Clinic — 213 604
Medical Director: Eli B. Mama, MD — 243 070

Kano

Iamat Center — Airport Road — 30 98 - 21 46
Co-ordinator: Albert Fahmy, MB, FRCP

NORWAY

Lillehammer

Skogli Badesanatorium — 51 513
Iamat Co-ordinator: Harold Lie, MD

OMAN

Muscat

Medident Centre
Medical Director: John R. H. Heap, MB, ChB, D.Obst. RCOG, MRCGP

PAKISTAN

Islamabad

Central Government Poly Clinic — 24 545 - 21 906
Medical Director: S. M. Malik, MD, MRCP (Glasg.), MRCP (Lond.)

Karachi

Karachi Adventist Hospital — 78 080 - 78 086
Medical Director: P. H. Tung, MD
Administrative Director: E. J. Johanson

Lahore

United Christian Hospital — 81 961/2 - 81 964
Medical Director: Immanuel Benjamin, MB, BS, MS, FRCS(C)
Administrative Director: John K. Mall

PANAMA

Colón

Hospital Samaritano — 471 780
Medical Director: Clemente P. Garnes, MD
Chief Nurse: Judith Chalhoub

Panama City

Clinica San Fernando — 237 453 - 616 666
Medical Director:
Ernesto Arosemena N., MD

Administrative Director: Teodoro Brin
Chief of Nursing:
Rosa E. de Batista
Iamat Co-ordinator:
Antoine Raymondo, MD 610 365 - 237 453

PAPUA NEW GUINEA

Boroko — Port Moresby

Iamat Center — Taumara Road 258 441 - 214 157
Co-ordinator:
Glen D. Mola, MD, MRCOG, DPH

Iamat Center — Tabari Place 253 353 - 253 701
Co-ordinator: George Chong Wah, MD

PERU

Lima

British American Hospital 403 570 - 409 100
(Clínica Anglo-Americana)
Medical Director:
Guillermo Garrido-Lecca, MD, FACC
Iamat Co-ordinator: Jaime Del Castillo, MD

PHILIPPINES

Bacolod

Bacolod Sanitarium and Hospital 26 631/2/3/4/5
Medical Director:
F. T. Geslani, MD, FPCS, FICS

Cebu

Miller Sanitarium and Hospital 75 833 - 94 581
Medical Director:
M. J. Tornilla, MD 97 004

Iligan City

Mindanao Sanitarium and Hospital 20 118
Medical Director: Levi Pagunsan, MD

Manila

Iamat Center — 1148 Roxas Blvd. or PAL Building — 595 256 - 501 487, 885 725
Co-ordinators: Luis A. Vazquez, MD
Danilo G. Jarina, MD
Juan G. Bailon, MD

Santiago — Isabela

Cagayan Valley Sanitarium and Hospital
Medical Director: Loreto Garcia, MD

POLAND

Warsaw

Iamat Center — Aleja Armii Ludowej 71-1 — 254 439 - 498 506
Co-ordinator: Prof. Witold J. Rudowski, MD, Hon. FACS

PORTUGAL

Cascais

Iamat Center — Av. Ultramar, 725 — 280 424
Co-ordinator: Josias Gyll, MD

Estoril

Iamat Center — Av. Marginal 11, — 260 775
Co-ordinator:
Armando Mendia D. Estrela, MD

Funchal - Madeira

Iamat Center — Avenida do Infante 26, "C" — 42 227, 33 292
Co-ordinator: Francis J. A. Zino, MD

Lagos

Casa de Saúde de Lagos — 63 026
Medical Director:
Manuel Rodrigues Clarinha, MD

Lisbon

Iamat Center — Rua Prof. Sousa da Câmara, 171-1 — 689 154, 651 213
Co-ordinator: Horácio da Silveira, MD

Iamat Center — Praça Olegario Mariano 6, 3rd floor left — 602 020, 821 747
Co-ordinator: Luis Teives, MD

Monte Estoril

Iamat Center — Avenida Saboia, 24 — 260 143 - 262 134
Co-ordinator: Aleixo Mariano de Souza, MD

Portimão

Iamat Center — Rua Machado San Ios — 312 2448 - 22 673
Co-ordinator: Estela Avellar de Castro, MD

Porto

Iamat Center — Rua de Santa Caterina 150 — 22 506
Co-ordinator: Pedro Ribeiro de Sousa Barbosa, MD — 680 221

Viana Do Castelo

Iamat Center — Rua Cândido dos Reis, 13–1.°–Esq. — 23 297
Co-ordinator: Gaspar Ferreira de Castro, MD

Viseu

Casa de Saúde de S. Mateus — 23 423/4/5
Medical Director: Luís Alberto Félix de Almeida Henriques, MD, SPRMN
Iamat Co-ordinator: Manuel de Sá Correia, MD, SPOG

PUERTO RICO

Mayagüez

Hospital and Policlinic Bella Vista — 832 2050
Medical Director: Benjamin A. Le Duc, MD — 832 2085
Administrative Director: Frank Perez
Iamat Co-ordinator: C. M. Donaldson, MD

Ponce

Hospital Damas — 843 5151
Medical Director: Ernesto Colón Yordán, MD
Executive Director: Héctor L. Sanchez

Vega Alta

Iamat Center — T. Ramirez 48 883 3155 - 883 3875
Co-ordinator: Ignacio J. Baez, MD

Vega Baja

Iamat Center — 8 Betances 858 2450
Co-ordinator: Raymond Báez Murphy, MD

RWANDA

Kigali

Iamat Center — In front of the Hotel Kiyovu 56 77
Co-ordinator: Ataullah Taaid, MD

SAMOA, AMERICAN

Pago Pago

Lyndon B. Johnson Tropical Medical Center 25 15

ST. LUCIA

Vieux Fort

St. Jude Hospital 60 41
Administrative Director: Sister Sharee Hurtgen

SAUDI ARABIA

Al-Khobar

Ash-Sharq Hospital 41 162 - 43 355 - 43 537
Medical Director: Joseph Yamin, MD

SCOTLAND

Aberdeen

Denburn Health Centre 20 952 - 30 997
Medical Director: Gordon Davidson Fraser, MBChB, MRCGP

Castlebay — Isle of Barra

Iamat Center 282
Co-ordinator: Robert D. Hill, MD

Edinburgh

Medical Centre — 19 Morningside Rd. 447 4139 - 447 4208
Iamat Co-ordinators:
W. H. Williams, MB, DRCOG
Alison Leach, MRCP UK, DCh

Elgin

Iamat Center — 12 Institution Rd. 75 12 - 77 15
Co-ordinator: Ernest Vincent C. Dawson, MB, FRCP

Falkirk

Iamat Center — 15 Booth Place 21 113
Co-ordinator: T. A. Wilson, MB, ChB

Fort William

Craig Nevis Surgery 29 47
Iamat Co-ordinator: Eric W. Irving, MB

Glasgow

Medical Centre — 311 Paisley Rd. W. 427 0191
Iamat Co-ordinators:
M. F. L. Barnes, MD
Brendan Sweeney, MB
George Barlow, MB

Iamat Center — 15, Whitehill Street 554 2989
Co-ordinator: Nathaniel Chazan, MB, ChB

Lerwick — Shetland Isles

Health Centre 32 01
Iamat Co-ordinators: E. A. Ingram, MB
R. B. Napier, MB
George Ewan, MB
R. Laidlaw, MB

Selkirk

Selkirk Health Centre 21 674
Iamat Co-ordinator:
Lindsay Douglas Neil, MB

SENEGAL

Dakar

Clinique Internationale 20 387 - 24 060 - 32 840
Medical Director:
Jean-Claude Bernou, MD

Iamat Center — 9, rue V. Hugo 216 848 - 226 530
Co-ordinator: Louis Leblanc, MD

SIERRA LEONE

Freetown

Iamat Center — Spiritus House, 8a
Howe Street 26 671
Co-ordinator: June Holst-Roness, MB, CHB (St. And.)

SINGAPORE

Singapore

Youngberg Memorial Adventist Hospital 889 271
Chief of Staff: Baldev Sing, MB, BS, MRCP
Administrative Director: J. A. Hay

SOUTH AFRICA, REPUBLIC OF

Cape Town

Die Volkshospital 226 755
Administrative Director: A. W. Truter

Johannesburg

Iamat Center — 501 Medical Towers 287 711
Co-ordinator: Joseph Teeger, MB, BCh 728 4298

SPAIN

Algeciras

Iamat Center — José-Antonio, 2 663 602 - 662 199
Co-ordinator: José L. Perales, MD

Caceres

Iamat Center — Avda. Virgen de Guadalupe 1 — 224 594 - 225 577
Co-ordinator: Silva Dominguez, MD

Gijon

Iamat Center — Alfredo Truán, 9-3.° Izda. — 341 435
Co-ordinator: Juán Dominguez García-Benito, MD

Lloret de Mar

Iamat Co-ordinator: Agustin Cabañas Llobet, MD — 364 067

Los Boliches — Fuengirola

Iamat Center — Avenida Los Boliches 76 — 474 347
Co-ordinator: Luis Alberro Rodriguez, MD

Madrid

The British American Hospital — 234 6700 - 233 3100
Medical Director:
Luis Rodriguez Fuentes
Iamat Co-ordinators: Eliseo M. Muñoz, MD
O. Saravalli,
J. M. Vidal, MD

Malaga

Clinica Santa Elena — 386 266 - 380 640
Iamat Co-ordinator: Mariano Martos, MD

Marabella

Iamat Center — Padre Enrique Cantos 5 — 772 396 - 772 492
Co-ordinator: Emilio Pino, MD

Palafrugell

Iamat Center — Plaza de España 8-2a — 300 135 - 300 931
Co-ordinator: José Bages Civill, MD

Pamplona

Clínica Universitaria — 255 400 - 255 900
University of Navarra
Medical Director: J. Cañadell, MD
Administrative Director: J. M. Paloma

Puerto de Pollensa (Balearic Islands)

Iamat Center 531 247 - 531 906
Co-ordinator: Andres Carretero Moya, MD

Reus

Iamat Center — Plaza Prim 5, 5 F 303 336 - 855 138
Co-ordinators: F. Moragas, MD
A. Morena, MD

San Antonio Abad (Ibiza)

Iamat Center — Calle Balanzat 1-1°-7 340 457
Co-ordinator: Arturo Ramos García, MD

San Sebastian

Hospital Provincial de San Sebastian 454 000
Medical Director: J. R. Ribera, MD 426 526 - 410 154
Technical Director of Hospital Services:
A. Olaso, MD

Santa Cruz de Tenerife (Canary Islands)

Iamat Center — Horazio Nelson 7 278 758
Co-ordinator: Tomas Zerolo Davidson, MD

Santander

Centro Médico Nacional "Marques de Valdecilla"
Head Cardiovascular Unit:
C. M. G. Duran, MD, D.PHIL

Seville

Iamat Center — Avda. El Greco 1 642 416
Co-ordinator: Patricio Brioso Vazques

Tolosa

Clínica Santa M. de la Asunción 661 941/2/3/4/5
Medical Director: J. R. Ribera, MD 426 526 - 410 154
Administrative Director: A. Izaguirre, MD

Torremolinos

Clínica Santa Elena 386 266 - 380 640
Iamat Co-ordinator: Mariano Martos, MD

Zaragoza

Clínica Quirurgica Montpellier — 239 359
Medical Director: Enrique Pelęgrin, MD
Iamat Co-ordinator: Fernándo Perlado, MD

SRI LANKA

Kandy

Lakeside Medical Center — 34 66
Medical Director: Merlyn E. Fernando, MD

SUDAN

Khartoum

The Khartoum Clinic — 44 479 - 44 133
Medical Director: W. Williams, MD, MRCS, LRCP, DKSM, MBBS
Administrative Director: Dardiry Mohamed Ahmed

SURINAME

Paramaribo

Iamat Center — Coesewijnestraat 3B Zorg en Hoop — 98 621
Co-ordinator: René Dawson, MD, MPH

Iamat Center — Weidestratt 60 — 72 653
Co-ordinator: F. J. C. Fung A. Foek, MD — 99 158

SWAZILAND

Mbabane

Mbabane Clinic Services — 24 25/6 - 28 86
Medical Director: Robin Stephenson, MD

SWEDEN

Göteborg

Iamat Center — Brämaregatan 11 — 220 011 - 224 432
Co-ordinator: Sven Hyllner, MD — 117 914

SWITZERLAND

Basel

Iamat Center — 42 Burgunderstrasse Co-ordinator: Martin Eisner, MD	234 934 - 478 533
Bethesda Spital Administrative Director: J. Buchmueller (Nonmember but cooperating hospital, not pledged to rate schedule.)	424 242

Bern

Iamat Center — Belpstrasse 11 Co-ordinator: Ed. Maibach, MD	252 040

Fribourg

Iamat Center — Rue St Pierre 28 Co-ordinator: PD Bernard C. Garnier, MD	221 414 - 220 506

Gland

Clinique La Lignière Medical Director: Christian P. Jaggi, MD, FMH	641 061

Lausanne

Clinique Cécil Medical Director: J. Rivier, MD Administrative Director: J. C. Salamin	201 251
Iamat Co-ordinator: Pierre Krieg, MD, FMH	236 665

Luzern

Klinik St. Anna Administrative Director: Sister Superior M. Th. Odermatt Iamat Co-ordinators: H. Fellmann, MD F. Gozon, MD E. Kopp, MD	301 133

Verbier

Polyclinic de Verbier Medical Director: A. Foletti, MD	74 024

Vevey

Iamat Center — Rue Hotel de Ville 17 Co-ordinator: Ulrich H. Schmid, MD	514 033 - 540 572

Iamat Center — Rue du Simplon 18 517 766 - 545 684
Co-ordinator: François Leu, MD
(For skin diseases only)

Zug

Kantonsspital Zug 231 344 - 216 534
Medizinische Abteilung
Medical Director: Prof. G. Keiser, MD

Zuerich

Iamat Center — Dolderstrasse 30 251 5229
Co-ordinator:
Claudia Sigg-Farner, MD, FMH

SYRIAN ARAB REPUBLIC

Banias

Clinique Médicale 234 437
Iamat Co-ordinator: Alexander Yazigi, MD

Damascus

Shifa Hospital 443 100 - 447 080
Medical Director:
Abdul Sattar Adi, MD, FACS 443 255
Administrative Director:
Ahmad Sawah, MD

TAHITI

Papeete

Clinique Cardella 28 190 - 29 708
Medical Director: Paul Zumbiehl, MD

TANZANIA

Serengeti National Park

Iamat members contemplating a safari in East Africa may obtain a tourist membership (fee $3.50) from the Flying Doctors' Society of Africa which offers ambulance flights in emergencies.

The Flying Doctors' Society of Africa
Nairobi, Kenya 27 281
Chairman: Mrs. Maddie De Mott

THAILAND

Bangkok

Iamat Center — Medi-Clinic, 968 Rama 4 Rd. 233 2533
Co-ordinator: Yong Uahwatanasakul, MD 286 1987

Bangkok Adventist Hospital 281 1422
Medical Director: Russel R. Standish, BA, MBBS, MRCP
Asst. Medical Director and Iamat Co-ordinator: Roland W. Brody, MBBS, FRACS

Chantaburi

Iamat Center — 89/1-2 Ampawa Road 311 521 - 311 030
Co-ordinator: Prakit Kasemsarn, MD

Chiengrai

Overbrook Hospital 311 366
Medical Director:
Kamphol Ongakasuvarn, MD

Haadyai

Haadyai Mission Hospital 243 599 - 243 139
Medical Director:
Raymundo Penaflorida, MD

Manorom (Chainat Province)

Manorom Christian Hospital
Medical Superintendent:
Peter R. Farrington, BDS, FDSRC
Iamat Co-ordinator:
G. Harverson, MRCP, FRCR

Nongbua (Nakonsawan Province)

Nongbua Christian Hospital
Medical Director:
Ursula Loewenthal, MB, ChB

Pattaya

Pattaya International Clinic 418 374/5
Iamat Co-ordinator:
Sunya Viravaidya, MB, BS (Melb.)

Songkhla

Songkhla General Hospital 311 494 - 311 017
Iamat Co-ordinator:
Lek Manomaiudom, MD, FICS 311 174

TONGA

Nuki'Alofa

Vaiola Hospital 200
Director of Health: Supileo Foliaki, MD
Medical Director: Opeti Jutui, MD

TRINIDAD

Port of Spain

Iamat Center — 46 Murray Street 22 544
Co-ordinator: Gordon A. Toby, MD

TUNISIA

Tunis

Iamat Center — 101 bis, Avenue de la Liberté 286 032 - 263 079
Co-ordinator:
Prof. M. Robbana, MD, FACS, FCCP 663 591 - 285 454

TURKEY

Adana

Iamat Center — Abidinpasa Caddesi, Kurttepeli Apt. Kat 1,
Co-ordinator: Muhittin Özbelli, MD 17 599 - 12 995

Ankara

Iamat Center — Necatibey Cad. 22/5 295 764 - 273 494
Co-ordinator: Osman Coskun, MD

Gaziantep

The American Hospital (Amerikan Hastahanesi) 10 69 - 34 20
Iamat Co-ordinator: Cemil Ozbal, MD

Istanbul

The Admiral Bristol Hospital 486 030
Medical Director: Warren H. Winkler, MD
Clinic Director: Ozkan Duygun, MD

Izmir

Fransiz Hastanesi (French Hospital) 33 934

UGANDA

Fort Portal

Virika Hospital 25 64
Medical Director: R. M. de Jong, MD

Kampala

Nsambya General Hospital 56 147 - 32 102
Medical Director: Johanna A. Cotter, MB BCh, MRCP (London)
Administrative Director:
Sister Louise Malone, SRN, SCM

URUGUAY

Montevideo

Hospital Britanico 406 022 - 409 011
Medical Director:
Jorge E. Stanham, MD, OBE
Administrative Director: Lars Torheim

VENEZUELA

Maracaibo

Centro Médico de Occidente 8 22 84 - 8 22 87
Medical Director:
Luís Maggiolo Atencio, MD

VIRGIN ISLANDS
St. Thomas

Charlotte Amalie

Knud Hansen Memorial Hospital — 774 1321 - 774 1212
Medical Director: Salvatore Tabacco, MD
Commissioner of Health:
Roy L. Schneider, MD, FACS, FICS
Administrative Director:
Mrs. Helen Banfield

St. Croix

Christiansted

Charles Harwood Memorial Hospital — 773 1311
Commissioner of Health:
Roy L. Schneider, MD, FACS, FICS
Assistant Commissioner:
Cora L. E. Christian, MD, MPH
Deputy Commissioner for Hospitals:
Lloyd K. Austin

YUGOSLAVIA

Belgrade

Interna Klinika B. Medicinkog Fakulteta — 685 922
Medical Director: Prof. V. Danilović
Administrative Director: M. Lalić
Iamat Co-ordinator: Vladan Josipović, MD

Dubrovnik

Medicinski Centar — 32 677
Medical Advisor: Prim. Branko John, MD — 27 712
Iamat Co-ordinator: Josip Rehak, MD — 22 677

Opatija

Institute for Treatment of Persons with Heart and Lung Diseases and Rheumatism — 712 322 - 722 500
Administrative Director:
Zlatko Perman, MD
Iamat Co-ordinator: Anton Oresković, MD

Split

Iamat Center — Lovretska 1/1 42 157
Co-ordinator: Zvonko Rumboldt, MD, PhD

Zadar

Medicinski Centar 24 677
Medical Director: Ante Gilić, MD
Iamat Co-ordinators:
Zelimir Mastrović, MD, MSPH
Martin Vabusek, MD

Zagreb

Zavod za bolesti srca — Rebro 213 948
(Heart Institute)
Medical Director:
Prof. R. Ivancić, MD, FACP 33 334
Iamat Co-ordinator: Assistant Prof. Z.
Asperger, MD, FACC 34 290

ZAIRE

Kinshasa

Iamat Center — Av. President
Tombalbaye 1286 22 300
Co-ordinators: Georges Dufays, MD
Mauro Forin, MD

Kisangani

Service Medical Sotexki 28 16
Medical Director:
Frederic Dalmau da Cruz
Administrative Director:
Mlle Babakwanza 31 53

Lubumbashi

Cliniques Universitaires Mama Mobutu 33 14
Medical Director:
Prof. Daniel Talleyrand, MD 29 40